BIRTH WITHOUT DOCTORS

BIRTH WITHOUT DOCTORS

JACQUELINE VINCENT-PRIYA

EARTHSCAN PUBLICATIONS LTD
LONDON

First published 1991 by
Earthscan Publications Ltd
3 Endsleigh Street, London WC1H 0DD

Copyright © Jacqueline Vincent-Priya 1991

British Library Cataloguing in Publication Data available

Designed by Sandie Boccacci
Production by Bob Towell
Typeset in 11/13 Janson by Rapid Communications Ltd, Bristol
Printed and bound by Guernsey Press

Earthscan Publications Ltd is an editorially independent
and wholly owned subsidiary of the International
Institute for Environment and Development (IIED)

CONTENTS

POSTSCRIPT

To

John Haggith

my father

and to my three daughters

Mary, Emma and Rachael

INTRODUCTION

IN 1986 I WENT to live in Malaysia with my partner Peter and our daughter Emma, who was then one year old. Peter had a job as a teacher and in the beginning I was anxious to find employment as a market researcher, as this was the work I had been doing for the previous twelve years in England. For the first six months I worked for a company in Kuala Lumpur but then, for reasons to do with the difficult state of the Malaysian economy, the job disappeared. Looking around for something to do, I decided that now would be a good time to research topics that were close to my heart rather than those that had commercial value. I had often thought about doing this, but because I had been so busy with a demanding career I had never before had the time. There seemed to be no shortage of interesting topics and it was some time before the subject of my work became clear.

Having recently given birth to Emma, I was interested in all aspects of pregnancy, birth and breastfeeding. I had found the experience of Emma's birth deeply fulfilling, both emotionally and spiritually, in contrast to the birth of my first daughter Mary, ten years previously. I was sure that one of the reasons why the birth had been so wonderful and why I had been able to manage without drugs was the support and encouragement I had received from my midwife, Anne. I still feel a very special affection for her when I think about Emma's birth and the things we experienced together.

At that time there had been several articles in the local Malaysian papers about traditional midwives. These were often extremely negative, but reading between the lines it

1

seemed that these practitioners gave women in labour the sort of help and support that I had received from Anne. I was intrigued and, with my Malaysian friend Ambi, arranged to go and talk to Buleh, the midwife described in the first chapter. This meeting affected me profoundly. I decided then and there that I wanted to find out more about these women who, until the recent introduction of Western medicine, were the main source of knowledge, help and support for women giving birth. In Malaysia traditional midwives were not allowed to practise freely and few young women were interested in acquiring this ancient wisdom. It seemed important to me to talk to traditional midwives before their knowledge disappeared for ever. One thing led to another and I widened my explorations to visit traditional midwives in different groups in both Thailand and Indonesia.

To find the midwives described in this book I travelled to various ethnic groups in the northern hills of Thailand and in different parts of Indonesia. The former journey I undertook during the four weeks of a Christmas holiday, and the latter during eight weeks of a summer vacation. The Malay and Orang Asli midwives I met on a number of short trips made to various parts of Malaysia. I visited so many groups that it was obviously impossible for me to become fluent in each of the languages, and I was therefore dependent mainly on Dang in Thailand and Letchumi in Malaysia and Indonesia to interview and translate for me. In each case we went together to the various villages, often staying there several nights so that we could not only find the midwife and talk to her but also experience a little of village life.

Travelling as a family with a young child did, I think, make us seem very non-threatening, especially when I started to breastfeed Emma, as this usually provoked a lot of interest. Once we had located the midwife – usually by asking someone who knew her to introduce us – I carefully explained what I was doing and asked if she would mind talking to me. Very few refused to do so, and many of the midwives were delighted that I was interested in their activities and was collecting this information so that it would not be forgotten. Most felt that they had something special to offer, particularly in terms of the spiritual powers which many of them felt they possessed. Despite the fact that I did not speak their language, lived in a completely different way and did not share their beliefs, I continued to be amazed at how close I felt to some of them. Our discussions about pregnancy and birth seemed to transcend all these differences and the feelings of closeness were often reciprocated. We taped most of the interviews (with their permission) and when we had finished I gave them a present. Sometimes this was money but sometimes it was the traditional present, maybe a sarong, which they would expect from a grateful client.

As a professional researcher I was well aware of the limitations of carrying out research in this way, but felt that within the financial and other constraints under which I worked I did the best that was possible. If I had waited for the resources to undertake the project "properly", I would never have got started. Having collected all the data, I thought long and hard about the best way of writing it up. I felt very strongly that I wanted not only to describe the information that these midwives gave me, but also to show the context in which they worked and from which their ideas and practices had grown. I also wanted to convey a sense of their personality, commitment and spirit, which had affected me so greatly when I met them. I decided that the best way of doing this was to write about and describe the women as I met them rather than analysing what they said out of the context in which they said it. In this way I hope that the women in these pages come across to you as individuals, in the same way that they did to me. I could not, of course, spend a very long time in each place, so I have used the work of other researchers to supplement my own impressions and to provide background information. I hope that, like me, you will be able to appreciate both the infinite variety and the similarities which these women share with each other and with us.

There are many, many people who have helped me with both the research and the writing of this book. I received a grant of M$2,000 from the Mentri Besar (chief executive) of Negeri Sembilan Datuk Hj. Mohd. Isa bin Datuk Hj. Abdul Samad DSNS.PMC. (I lived in Seremban, the capital of the state of Negeri Sembilan, for the four years I spent in Malaysia.) I also received M$2,000 from the Malaysian Culture Group in Kuala Lumpur. These two grants enabled me to travel to Indonesia and to pay Letchumi for all her work there. I was very grateful indeed for this support, as not only did it considerably ease my financial situation but at the time it also gave me a very necessary psychological boost. A special thanks must go to Dang and to Letchumi, who between them did the bulk of the interviewing and translating. Both of them were wonderful travelling companions. Other people who have helped include Judy Moody-Stuart, who gave me a lot of encouragement as well as suggesting that I apply for a grant from the Malaysian Culture Group. She also lent us her four-wheel-drive vehicle so that we could visit some Orang Asli villages in the remoter parts of the jungle. Writing a book is always a somewhat isolating exercise, especially when there are few friends living nearby with whom to talk. Chris Corrin, Paul Kitchener, David Fairhurst and Eddie Heaton-Smith all wrote to me regularly and were a great source of support through the particularly lonely times. Special thanks must go to Peter, who has been with me since the genesis of this book and has supported me both financially and emotionally as it has grown and evolved. Finally, a very special thanks to the midwives who shared themselves and their knowledge so generously with me. This is their book as much as mine.

1
꿔꿩

IN THE BEGINNING . . .

ACCORDING TO THE local Malaysian newspapers, traditional midwives like Buleh are a very bad thing. Their
ignorance and insanitary techniques are the main cause of
higher maternal and infant mortality in rural areas. They are
the cause of problems like premature delivery, mental handi-
cap and ruptured uterus. They carry out abortions which are
illegal and unsafe. If only mothers would be sensible enough
not to use their services, and use the government midwives
instead, such problems would be a thing of the past.

What the writers of these articles never mention, of course,
is that the people living in rural areas are poorer, with
larger families, and are less well nourished than the rest of
the population. This could equally well explain the higher
mortality rates, although no one has ever collected the sort
of information which would show the real causes. Putting
the blame on traditional midwives conveniently absolves the
authorities from acknowledging this poverty, and covers up
what I later found were glaring inadequacies in the medical
services provided in rural areas. These articles also never
pointed out the more questionable practices in the local hospitals and clinics. Many hospitals have a conveyor-belt system
for mothers who are giving birth, with routine intervention
and no facilities for fathers or other family members to provide

support. Figures are difficult to come by, but there are some hospitals which have an episiotomy rate of nearly 100 per cent, and a high rate of Caesarean deliveries. In many places there is routine separation of mother and child immediately after birth and a consequent very low rate of breastfeeding. Traditional midwives may have their inadequacies, but so too do the government hospitals and private clinics.

Whatever the papers said about traditional midwives, I couldn't help but have a sneaking affinity for them. They were, after all, part of a long line of women who had been helping other women give birth long before the advent of modern medicine, and in many parts of the world are still the main source of help for pregnant and labouring mothers. Although some of their practices might be questionable and their ability to cope with serious complications limited, they surely could not be all bad. Did women give birth successfully because of them or in spite of them? Many of my local friends used a traditional midwife, if not for the birth then to massage and care for them afterwards, and had been very satisfied with the help they had received. The more I heard about them, the more I wanted to meet and talk with them; to find out for myself what they were like, how they learnt their craft and what they did to help women in labour, birth and afterwards.

I had had plenty of research experience, but the techniques I had used to find respondents in England clearly wouldn't work when it came to finding a traditional midwife in Malaysia. They usually live in tight-knit rural communities which are difficult for an outsider, especially a foreign outsider, to penetrate. There was also the language problem; the official language of Malaysia is Bahasa Malaysia but various Chinese dialects, Tamil and English are also extensively spoken, and beneath these hide many of the diverse dialects found amongst the different language groups. Buleh, for instance, spoke her own dialect which, although like Bahasa Malaysia, contained many of its own unique expressions and words.

For these reasons I found myself involved with what was to become a familiar pattern. First I would find someone who knew the midwife well and was willing to come with me and introduce me to her. The first time this "someone" was Arifin, an old Chinese man who had married and divorced a Malay wife many years ago and now lived on his own in a small and very bare wooden house in a field behind some shophouses in the small town of Tanjong. His simple life was spent growing coconuts and acquiring the little money he required to satisfy his basic needs. Helping me was for him an interesting diversion from the coffee shop where he spent most of his time and where we met before going to see Buleh.

The coffee shop was part of a row of old wooden shophouses, the sort of building you find all over Malaysia. It consisted of a terrace of shops along the bottom, which were open to the pavement, and small living quarters above. We sat at tables which, I was amused to see, were just like the tables found in many of the more pretentious pubs and wine bars which I used to frequent in my market research days – large curly legs made of cast iron topped with a huge slab of marble. These, like the cracked cups from which we drank our coffee, must have been the original furniture which was bought 100 or 150 years ago when the shop was first opened. The walls were festooned with dusty plaques on which Chinese characters had been engraved, and there were a number of large, heavy, glass-fronted cabinets filled with a miscellaneous selection of objects which I presume could have been sold but looked as if they hadn't been touched for years. Out the back a tall Chinese in shorts slowly poured a brown liquid from one pot to the other, making the "tea tariq", which means literally "pulled tea". This tea, which is made with condensed milk, is poured from one pot to another to make it frothy, and can look rather like espresso coffee. We sat sipping our drinks and listening to the birds screeching and flying up and down to their nests, which were just under the eaves of the shop roof.

Buleh lived in the village of Talang, about three miles along a winding country road outside Kembang. Her house was situated at the top of a steep bank overlooking the flat rice fields where the villagers grew most of their own rice. Steps had been cut into the bank and a variety of bottles, stones and pieces of wood had been used to make a sturdy staircase. Overhanging plants kept the steps shady and cool in the humid atmosphere, and I blinked as we emerged into the bright sunlight at the top to meet Buleh and her husband, whose first action was to show us their singing stones. According to them, the stones used to sing regularly, making a humming noise and sometimes chanting verses from the Koran, but for some reason in the last few years they hadn't done so. Having just arrived, I found this very odd, but by the time I left and had come to appreciate Buleh's conception of the universe, it didn't seem at all peculiar.

Buleh was dressed in the traditional Malay way, with a batik sarong tied around her waist and worn with a loose top. She said she was in her late fifties or maybe early sixties, and with her quick smile I liked her immediately. She seemed to exude a quiet confidence and there was an incredible feeling of calm and positivity around her. She said that she felt she had something special to offer mothers who came to her for help, and seemed very pleased that I had come to talk to her. She showed us into her spacious wooden house which was built in the local style, on stilts. As this sort of design allows the air to circulate all around the house, it was deliciously cool even on this very hot and humid day. There I met Buleh's daughter Rahimah, who was sitting breastfeeding her three-month-old daughter Rosanah, Buleh's latest grandchild, whom she had helped to deliver and of whom she was extremely proud.

Buleh took us into the kitchen, where she was boiling some herbs to give to her daughter. They looked like a bundle of small sticks tied together and were simmering in a large pan of water. They are known as *akar kayu*, and according to Buleh these herbs are taken by all mothers during their confinement period, usually for at least three days after giving birth, although Rahimah took it for a full forty-four days. Buleh said she knew the names of all the herbs used and that she collected them from the jungle herself. "The *akar kayu* is not only useful for women in childbirth but can be used by anyone wishing to strengthen their internal organs. We Kampong people say that it is good for diabetes, high blood pressure and various other ailments. For new mothers the herbs strenghten the womb and bring the body back to normal." I tried the herbs – they had a not unpleasant but not very distinctive taste, and made me sweat slightly. According to Buleh, this would help to get rid of toxins in the body. These herbs can now be bought as tablets, and later I found other midwives who used them in this form; but not Buleh – she thought the ones she gathered herself from the jungle were far superior.

As we sat drinking the herbs I asked Buleh how she had become a midwife – or *bidan*, as she is called by the Kampong people: "I have been working as a *bidan* on my own for about fifteen years, but I was quite young when I started helping my mother, who was the *bidan* here before me. I helped massage pregnant women and also sprained muscles and that sort of thing. It was only after my mother died that I took over this work completely on my own. My mother was a *dukun* [a kind of traditional doctor who uses both herbal and spiritual methods to cure disease] and she was used to the spirit world. Many people knew her and came to her for help, and she was carrying on a tradition that had been handed down in our family for generations. After my mother died she appeared to me in a dream and instructed me to place a yellow-coloured dress under my pillow. She told me to wear it for a few days and then she would come to me again in my dreams. This she did, and I realized that she was my guardian spirit, the one who used to be with my mother, and that now my mother had died she was passing on to me. Oh no! I was never scared of the spirit, for it always appeared in the form of my mother and it has accepted me as its grandchild."

Buleh felt very close to her spirit, and spoke about her as if she were another member of the family. As I sat and listened to her, it didn't feel at all strange or odd that she should be in contact with the supernatural in this way, and it was also important to the women who came to her for help. Arifin told us afterwards that Buleh is a much-respected midwife in the village, not only for the practical help she provides but also for the spiritual power she can draw on if there are any problems. As Buleh's spirit gives her confidence, so it also gives confidence to her clients.

As Buleh said, however, the spirit won't go to just anyone: "The spirit is very choosy and selects only those who it feels are honest with no malice in their hearts. The spirit instructs me to be pure-hearted in my dealings, never to take revenge and to do good to others. We believe that the spirit is a messenger from Allah [she described it as like a Muslim saint, whom she referred to as a *wali*] who can do only good to people." Buleh had great confidence in the help her spirit would provide, having experienced this in the past: "I still have contact with the spirit; whenever we are in difficulties the spirit will help us by telling us to keep calm, not to worry and be patient. When anyone is giving birth I only have to call on the spirit, who will show me what to do. To lessen the pain of childbirth I sometimes massage very gently, but if the pain is very bad then I appeal to the guardian spirit. I use the water of a young coconut, over which I chant some prayers so that the guardian spirit enters the water. When the mother drinks the water, then the spirit gets into the body and helps her with the birth. No, I cannot reveal the special prayers that I use, as these are confidential between me and the spirit. I always give mothers this special water before the baby is born."

Similarly, she was able to ask for the help of the spirit for more serious problems: "If during the birth the feet of the child appear first, we use prayers to right the problem; I have never had any difficulties with this sort of birth. We request the help of the guardian spirit, who gets Allah's help to right the problem." In some cases she felt that her methods were at least as good as those available in the hospitals: "There was a case I attended where doctors had said the head was in the wrong position. I said some prayers over some water and made the patient drink it. After that the baby moved by itself into the right position."

After telling me this, however, Buleh was quick to point out that these techniques were used "in the old days", before the advent of the present medical system which included government midwives trained in Western techniques: "These days there are strict laws to abide by, and government midwives have to be present at every birth. Of course if the baby arrives unexpectedly then we will attend, but at the same time we must call for the government midwife. She does not live nearby, and if she is busy with another birth we have to look for another one. We have to wait for her, as now there are very strict rules about what we *bidans* can do. Nowadays," Buleh said, if any sort of complications developed, she sent the women to hospital: "Even if there is not time to send to the hospital I would not dare to do anything because of the government restrictions on unregistered midwives; we must follow the law. We just massage now, so our work is much easier."

I was very surprised to learn that Buleh did not necessarily see the women she helped in labour and birth during their pregnancy. According to her, it all depended on whether the women felt that they needed to see her or not. Often they would come near the beginning of a pregnancy to check whether they were pregnant or to find out whether the baby was growing properly and in the right position for birth. In this village, however, that did not mean a woman would be isolated in her pregnancy, as she might be if she lived in England or America. With a very strong social network, a pregnant woman would have the support of her other female relatives and friends, who would keep an eye on her and give her any help and advice she wanted. As Buleh explained: "In those days the hospital was far and it was too difficult to send the patient there, but then we rarely had birth complications. This is because we had taken all the precautions to get the mother ready for birth while she was pregnant. We made sure that she was healthy and there were no problems, so normally we didn't have to face any complications. Now if there are complications I leave it to the government midwife to handle."

Untrained personnel are not allowed to cut the umbilical cord, "because we don't have the right instruments to do it", but Buleh showed me how she used to do it. This was obviously another important ritual aspect, as she put a special black scarf round her head as she did so: "In the old days *bidans* used to cut the umbilical cord themselves using a piece of bamboo. First I massage the umbilical cord to pacify the baby. Then we put the silver coin and a slice of turmeric under the cord and the cord is then cut with the bamboo." I loved the way she was so thoughtful for the babies; are they aware of the cord being cut? Do they feel anything? This isn't something I have ever heard discussed amongst Western practitioners. Both the bamboo and the turmeric have antiseptic qualities, and of course in this context they also have the advantage of being very easily available and disposable after use, thus probably cutting down on infection.

Despite having a government midwife service with strict laws about what *bidans* can and cannot do, there is no follow-up for mothers as there is, for instance, in the United Kingdom, with the midwife calling regularly to see that both mother and baby are well. Perhaps, then, it is just as well that one of the most important things Buleh does is the massage for mothers after they have given birth, together with teaching about breastfeeding (if they need it) and looking after the baby. Most Malay women are very concerned to have massage after birth, as they believe that this is the best way not only of recovering their pre-pregnancy shape but also of ensuring that all their bodily organs, particularly the uterus, go back to their original size and position. I was delighted when Buleh asked if I would like to watch her massaging Rahimah. I had assumed that this would be very difficult to see, as Malay women tend to be very shy, even in front of other women, and I could hardly believe my luck when the first person I talked to was willing to do it.

Buleh began by preparing the binding for the stomach by taking a few handfuls of ash from the smoking fire. She placed them on a piece of newspaper, then took two small onions and a piece of garlic. Holding them in her hands, she said some prayers, after which she cut the onions and garlic up into the ash without peeling them. She rolled the newspaper into a small bundle which she could hold easily in her hand, took a piece of white cotton cloth about two yards long, knotted one end of it and tucked the newspaper parcel into it. Taking the binding, Buleh showed us into the bedroom where Rahimah, in her sarong, was waiting to be massaged although, as she explained, after the birth she

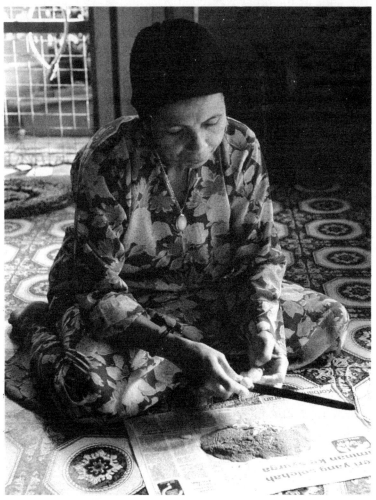

Cutting garlic and onions into the ash used in preparing the binding

would first have had a special bath in which the water would be mixed with herbs to help her feel fresh and energetic.

As she massaged her daughter, Buleh told us about the oil she used and how she made it up herself from coconuts. Each client was massaged differently, according to her needs: "I learn the method of massage from my dreams. What I do is not the same as the other Kampong *bidans*, as every one of us has her own methods. With different mothers I do the massage in various ways because each person needs something different. How do I know what to do? Well! I just know; I learn from my dreams. The spirit has shown me how to massage to increase the milk flow [she did this by putting oil on Rahimah's back and rubbing with her thumbs on both sides of her shoulders]. Massaging the legs and thighs like this is like exercise; you get the same results. The massage makes the body supple and brings back lost vigour. After the massage I give them *akar kayu*."

When it came to the stomach, Buleh massaged the sides with the oil and then pressed the womb up before placing the rolled bundle of ash mixture right under it. She then wound the remaining cloth around the stomach to keep the bundle in place. The stomach was bound tightly, and to finish another piece of material was tied round; this had cords on it and kept the bandage in place. Rahimah, who had had this treatment for a month after birth, had a beautiful flat stomach and there was no sign that it had ever been distended with pregnancy: "For forty-four days a woman has to wear the binding. It is taken off when she has a bath and is put back on again after the massage. We wear it even in bed." Buleh finished by combing oil through Rahimah's hair: "When I comb the hair with oil this helps to improve eyesight and keeps the skin looking supple and youthful."

As the baby was awake, Buleh said she would show us how she bathed her. She began by preparing a mixture of limes (picked from the tree which grew just outside her house), rice flour and water, cutting up the limes into small pieces and mixing them together with water and her special silver coin. As she mixed the ingredients she recited some special prayers over them. Again, she wouldn't tell us exactly what these were, but said that they were special Muslim prayers for

14

this particular activity. The baby was then bathed with some plain water and the mixture was poured over her, after

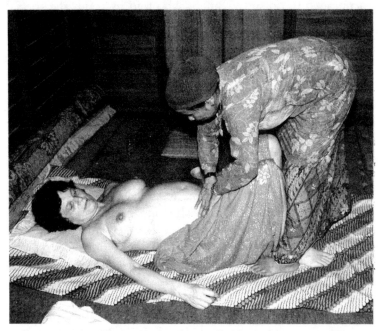

The author being massaged by Buleh

which she was wiped dry. Buleh used tapioca flour all over the baby's body to keep her cool and help reduce rashes from prickly heat. I noticed that they also had a pot of Johnson's baby powder, but I really couldn't see the point when the traditional tapioca flour was so fine and soft and didn't contain additives like perfume; but I suppose that's progress – or is it?

Buleh's husband then showed us how he said prayers for the baby just after she was born. Getting out his prayer mat and facing it towards Mecca, he held the baby and recited some prayers for her. The baby's father wasn't at home for the birth (he is in the army) so this was done by the grandfather, although it could also be done by either the father or the grandmother. After the birth of a baby there isn't a special celebration apart from these prayers, although Rahimah told us that they have a special ceremony during the seventh month of pregnancy and three months after the baby is born. Rahimah was breastfeeding, having been strongly encouraged to do so by Buleh, who told us about the special ritual they have before the baby is breastfed for the first time (usually immediately after the bath and prayers): "After the baby is bathed we bring it to the mother to be fed, but before it is fed for the first time we rub a little salt on its lips, and then some gold. This is our Malay tradition."

Apart from helping mothers in childbirth, Buleh also helped with other "women's problems" like infertility and contraception; she has herbs to help both problems and, despite government contraception being widely available, is still in demand for this service. We asked her about abortion, but as it is illegal in Malaysia (especially for Muslims) she wasn't willing to say whether she did this or not. Afterwards Arifin told me that most country people know of ways of procuring an abortion, one of them being to put the sap found in a very common grass into their uterus. Apparently this is supposed to work well, provided it is done early enough in the pregnancy.

And payment for her services? Like almost all the midwives I eventually went on to meet, Buleh sees what she is doing as a social service rather than a professional-type job: something she does for the community over and above the necessary rice-growing and other work which she needs to do to live: "I do get paid for my work as a *bidan*, but the amount is left to them. I don't demand the payment because some of my patients are poor people. If they don't have the money, how are they going to pay me?"

I suppose Buleh lived no more than twenty miles or so from the town where I lived – which, with its shops, banks and people going about their business, is much like a town anywhere. Yet in that relatively short physical distance I felt I had come a much further distance psychologically. As we drove back home and "normality" reasserted itself, I felt as if Buleh had taken me into a special sort of glasshouse where, for just a little while, I had been able to look out and see my normal world transformed. For Buleh, giving birth was part of a woman's identity: a normal event which, although it had its dangers, usually proceeded without difficulties. For me, giving birth was not an inevitable event or part of my identity as a woman, but a conscious choice arrived at after a certain amount of agonizing. My experience of birth had been very mixed, but I still viewed it as something unusual and more likely to go wrong than right. I was also surprised at the centrality to Buleh's work of the spiritual aspect which of course, in the Western context, has been lost beneath a plethora of hi-tech gadgets. It is very easy to dismiss Buleh's spirituality as so much mumbo jumbo which can't possibly do any good, yet it gave considerable confidence to both her and her clients. Who is to say that this confidence, wherever it comes from, does not help women give birth or deal with difficulties? Clearly Buleh would be unable to deal with the sort of problems which require surgical or other intervention, but even Western doctors accept that this applies to only a very small proportion of women.

On the practical side, there seemed to be so many questions that needed answering. Do all traditional midwives learn what to do as Buleh did, from her mother? What sort of things did they do to help women give birth? Would we be able to use any of this in the West? How were traditional midwives thought of and treated in the villages where they lived and worked? Was the spiritual aspect always so strong and important? Why couldn't their experience and talents be used in the overall healthcare system rather than, as in Buleh's case, being ignored completely? There and then I decided that as long as we lived in this part of the world where traditional midwives still live and work, I would talk to more of them and try to answer some of these questions.

For the next two years I travelled around different parts of South-East Asia and talked to both mothers and midwives in different ethnic groups. While I did formulate some answers to the questions that I had initially set myself, time and again I found myself looking at and sometimes feeling part of what

I can only describe as another kind of reality. Looked at as a purely physical process, giving birth is the same for women everywhere, and in the West we probably think we know more about it than ever before in our history. For the woman giving birth, however, the process is viewed in many different ways according to how she perceives herself both individually and as part of the group in which she lives. It was tapping this rich vein of women's experience of birth which I found most interesting. It involved looking not only at the practical ways in which women help each other to labour and give birth, but also at the context in which this event took place. Often this meant examining what some call "non-ordinary reality" or "intuition" and the ways in which women viewed themselves as part of the larger cosmos, sometimes described as "their religious world-view". To understand these things, it seemed to me, required an understanding of the total context of these women's lives, and to describe their experiences outside this context would be to do an injustice to what they had told me.

This book is not, therefore, an analysis of different systems of giving birth or a series of case studies which set out to answer questions or prove a point. Rather, it is a kaleidoscope of different birth experiences put within the context of the lifestyle and beliefs of the women who experienced them. I made the physical journey to different and sometimes fairly outlandish places, talking to mothers and midwives. At the same time I found myself making an internal journey through my ideas and emotions which brought me to my own knowledge about giving birth and which I found, when I became pregnant for the third time, had changed me profoundly.

PART I

TREKKING IN
THAILAND

2

Into Northern Thailand

THE PREVIOUS YEAR we had visited Changmai in Thailand, where we had first come into contact with people from what are loosely called the "hill tribes". These are a collection of different ethnic groups, each of which has its own very distinctive language, dress, religion and lifestyle. Even in cosmopolitan Changmai they couldn't help but stand out, with their colourful clothes and independent manner. There are thought to be around 500,000 of them (out of a total Thai population of about fifty million) living in small villages which are scattered over the most inaccessible hills of the twenty-one northern provinces.

In the last few years a considerable trekking industry has grown up around Changmai, with tourists being taken to stay at hill tribe villages, but despite this onslaught, most of these groups continue with their traditional way of life. We were extremely lucky in meeting Dang, who had taken us trekking during our first visit to this area. I had enjoyed going with him immensely, as he seemed to be genuinely interested in and friendly with the villagers, and to accept their way of living readily. With him I had felt less of a tourist than I might have done, and that I had actually experienced, even for a very short while, living in another lifestyle rather than just coming and staring at it from the outside. When I thought about where

I could go to meet more traditional midwives, these isolated villages seemed like good places. Even those living in the more accessible communities were rarely in a position where they could get to a doctor or hospital easily, so they had to depend on themselves to deal with things like childbirth and most of the medical problems they might encounter. As the different groups had such distinctive lifestyles, I was also hoping that I would be able to see a range of different ideas and practices in a reasonably short time.

Ever since the previous year I had therefore been in contact with Dang, explaining what I wanted to do and asking him to make all the necessary local arrangements. This did not always go as smoothly as I'd hoped, as Dang seemed to spend his time between his home in Changrai and his workplace in Changmai. Sometimes it would take several letters to the two different places before I received a long and apologetic letter in reply. As we were going to be talking to women about a subject which might be seen only as a women's concern, I thought it essential to have one or more women to interpret for me. This is harder to set up than it might seem, as there are few women who have the necessary experience with all the different languages, and of these only a few are or would want to become involved with trekking. Whatever the difficulties, however, Dang was optimistic that he could find the female help I needed.

Returning to Changmai was like returning home, even after a hair-raising bus drive through the flood-torn south. This was just after the devastating floods in 1988, when many hundreds of people had been killed and rail links were completely severed for a while. Once I had arrived in Bangkok, the rest of the journey was carried out in much better style on the train which goes nightly from the capital to Changmai. After the overwhelming size and noise of Bangkok I was very pleased to arrive in Changmai, which always feels more like a city on a human scale. It does have its own traffic problems, but somehow it always seems easier here to escape from them to the small back lanes away from the main roads, which are usually more peaceful.

Dang once again seemed very elusive, and I wondered if he'd been in the right place to receive my last letter telling him of the date of my arrival. After some fruitless phone calls and running around to his various haunts in Changmai, I finally managed to track him down to sort out the final details. It seemed there were some problems. Despite Dang's optimism, in the end none of the female interviewers could be persuaded to come, as the one or two who did this sort of work were too busy in this, the main tourist season. Dang, however, could see no problem with doing the interviews himself. Well – to be fair, he could see why there could be a problem, but thought that given his relationship with the villagers, there wouldn't actually be one! I wasn't very happy about it, but at this late stage couldn't see any alternative. Getting the resources together for this trip had not been easy, and every day of delay was costing me money; I certainly didn't have the resources or time to spend too long waiting for someone to turn up, and learning all the necessary languages myself was obviously out of the question. As usual I had to balance what was feasible against what in a perfect world would be desirable, and decided it was better to go ahead and get something rather than nothing. So despite my misgivings I decided that Dang would do the interviewing, which turned out much better than I probably had any right to expect.

Emma, my daughter, was only three years old at the time, so the distances she could walk were very limited. I felt we couldn't go to really remote places, some of which required a trek of a day or more on foot. We therefore decided to confine ourselves to villages where there was not more than an hour or two's walking from a road. These villages wouldn't be "untouched", but we hoped their inhabitants would still be living a fairly independent lifestyle unaffected by the worst ravages of tourism. We also had someone to help us carry Emma when she got tired - the seventeen-year-old son of the van driver. He was a very personable young man who cheerfully fitted in with everything we did and who, I was very surprised to learn, had been having considerable problems at school. He was apparently very intelligent but had got in with a group taking drugs and had been missing a lot of his schoolwork. His father had brought him on this trip in an attempt to keep more of an eye on him, hoping that he would eventually calm down and could be sent to a different school where he would be more likely to manifest some of his academic potential.

Having organized the trip, there was nothing more to do for a few days except enjoy Changmai and all that it had to offer. I found it rather unnerving that Dang had gone home again, with his beautiful French girlfriend Pascale, and was impossible to contact. I kept thinking of things I wanted to ask and things I wanted to check up, but as there was no opportunity for this I had no option but to calm my restless mind and enjoy the civilized delights of Changmai while I had the chance. There was nothing to do but sit and wait and, as so often happens in this part of the world, allow events to unfold rather than make them happen.

On the morning of our journey we wondered whether all our worst fears were going to materialize when the time for departure came and went. Eventually Pascale turned up without Dang, who had apparently had difficulty in securing sleeping bags and was running around Changmai trying to find some alternatives. We went and did some shopping which included medical supplies, as we had thought that we might have some medical students with us. Unfortunately they couldn't come but as the villagers, who had been warned of our coming, were expecting doctors, Dang thought it as well to take something in the medical line. We could, of course, have bought all manner of powerful Western drugs at the local chemist, but given my predilection for more natural remedies we made do with paracetamol and Dettol as probably being the least innocuous – always provided they were taken sensibly, which couldn't of course be guaranteed.

As we drove out of Changmai, my lively mind was in direct contrast to the flat scenery all around. At this time of the year it was warm, but not excessively so, with fresh mornings and clear blue skies. As we drove past the flat rice fields we could see people bringing in what looked like a very good harvest. Not having had time to buy provisions at the supermarket in Changmai, we stopped at Hod to visit the shop of a friend of Dang's. This turned out to be the most sundry sundry shop I have ever visited, with a very wide range of dusty tins and packets of this and that cluttering the shelves. What she didn't actually have on the shelves she obtained from various other shops around. We bought vegetables, and Dang bought a piece of pork as a present for the person with whom we were going to stay in the village. Fortunately at that time I did not know how it was going to be eaten – chopped up raw with herbs!

Gradually the countryside became more and more hilly as we went deeper into hill tribe territory until we finally swung off the road and bumped up the track to visit our first village.

MOTHERS AS MIDWIVES:
WITH THE LAHU
IN NORTHERN THAILAND

ON THE NARROW bumpy track which led to the Lahu
village of Pon Nyi our small van had to pull into the side
three times to let bus loads of tourists go by. When we finally
arrived at the village two other buses were disgorging their
passengers, who immediately began milling around and taking
photographs with cameras of greater or lesser sophistication.
One person, sporting a video camera of such size that it needed
to be carried around on his shoulder, was pointing it at a rather
disconsolate child carrying a baby who was, it seemed, quite
impervious to his requests for some sort of reaction that he
could record on his film.

As we got out of our van we were besieged by children
begging for sweets, and Thai *baht* to have their picture taken.
Their whining, piercing cries contrasted strangely with their
bubbling, satisfied laughter when they managed to extract
anything from the visitors. I was horrified, as I couldn't
believe that this daily invasion was not affecting the villagers'
lifestyle. Dang, however, seemed quite unmoved as he told
me matter-of-factly about the realities of the tourist business:
"There are some hot springs on the main road nearby and a
lot of tourist buses go there. As these people want to see a
primitive village and this one isn't far off the road, they stop
here so they can have a look. But no one ever stays here, so

the villagers just go on living as they always have."

As I later found, this was true up to a point. Although there was a steady stream of tourists, few ventured into the village beyond the houses near where the buses stopped. They also stayed a very short time, generally no more than five minutes or so. The worst effect, I found, was the distorted image that each group had of the other. As the tourists came to the village to see something primitive, so the villagers, especially the children, saw the tourists as rich people to exploit to the utmost. As Dang said, however, no one had ever stayed in the village before, and when he said that we were going to do so this caused tremendous excitement. A group of children rushed off to inform others in the village, while a small posse of them came with us to show the way, talking excitedly to Dang as we slowly walked to the headman's house.

There was nothing to distinguish this house from all the others, and as we climbed on to the low platform we were met by Nargat, the headman's wife, breathless from her exertions of sweeping the house out in readiness for our arrival. She looked rather careworn and I thought at first she would be very shy, but she made us feel very welcome and, I found later, wasn't the least intimidated by us.

The house was made completely of bamboo and stood on short stilts. We stepped from the veranda into one of the two window-less rooms where needles of sunlight coming through the split bamboo walls pierced the dusty dimness. The floor was also made of split bamboo and creaked alarmingly as we walked across it. I felt I could easily put my foot through its seemingly fragile construction. Eventually I found that the only way to walk around comfortably was *not* to look at my feet and to imagine that the floor was made of something more substantial, like wooden planks. These floors have a lot of advantages: they are cool, and dirt and other debris can easily be pushed through the slats to the ground below where, provided it is edible, the pigs, chickens and dogs will clean it all up.

As we sat on the veranda enjoying the evening, a steady stream of visitors came to have a good look at us, including

many children who were fascinated by Emma and wanted
to touch her blonde hair. They were very welcoming and
it wasn't long before Emma was playing their games, one of
which involved pretending to husk and winnow rice using
a very small flat basket and stones which were tossed up
into the air. Many of the children were carrying younger
brothers and sisters who looked large enough to be almost
the same age as themselves. Several young mothers, who I
later heard were only about fourteen or fifteen, came up to
have a look while they proudly displayed their breastfeeding
babies.

Originally the Lahu are thought to have come from Tibet,
and to have migrated over the centuries to the southern
provinces of China. Here they stayed until the eighteenth
or nineteenth century, when large numbers moved out to
Burma and Laos as a result of political upheavals in China.
As the need for more farming land increased they moved
further south, and in the first decades of the twentieth century
came into Thailand. Since then the unrest in both Burma and
Laos and the relatively peaceful existence in Thailand have
encouraged many more Lahu to move there. They are one of
the smallest of the hill tribe groups with a population which
has been estimated at between 16,000 and 40,000, although
smaller estimates are probably more correct. This accounts
for only about 6 per cent of the Lahu, most of whom still
continue to live in the surrounding countries of China, Burma
and Laos.

Dang told me about the different groups of Lahu: "There
are four groups, known as the Lahu Nya (Red Lahu), Lahu
Na (Black Lahu), Lahu Sla (Yellow Lahu) and Lahu Shele
(Lahu of Unknown Origin). As you can see, this village is
Black Lahu because all their clothes are black, but if you
go to the villages of the other groups their clothes will be
different colours." This seemed a reasonable assumption given
my experience of this village and of the Red Lahu village we
subsequently visited, where clothes were predominantly red.
This is not apparently always the case, however, and I later
found that the colours have a deeper symbolism. The groups

keep themselves quite distinct and tend to live and marry within the group.

Before it grew dark we decided to have a closer look at the village. With a small group of children excitedly dancing about us we walked around the houses, picking our way carefully over the rough ground and avoiding all the pigs, chickens and dogs that were running around freely. Lahu villages usually consist of fifteen to twenty-five houses

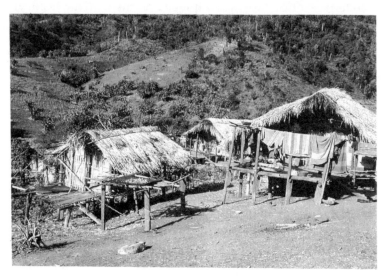

The Black Lahu village

so this one was very large, with more than forty houses and about two hundred inhabitants. As the headman told us later, "We've been here about ten years and when we moved everyone moved together as we wanted to find better land on which to grow [opium] poppies." Realizing that he might have been rather tactless, he quickly modified this last remark: "Of course nowadays most of our income comes from growing rice and corn rather than from growing poppies." The Thai government has tried very hard to encourage the opium-growing hill tribes to grow something else, but of course it is extremely difficult to think of a crop which would provide anything like the income derived so easily from opium poppies. Traditionally, the Lahu are "pioneer" swidden cultivators, burning a patch of jungle which they cultivate for a few years until the soil is exhausted, and then moving on. Nowadays there is little or no land left for this type of agriculture and many villages carry out lowland types of cultivation, including irrigated rice. Generally the main subsistence crops are dry hill rice, buckwheat and maize, with opium and chillies being grown for cash.

Modern realities have also impinged on the way the headman of the village is now chosen, as Nargat's husband explained: "In the past the whole village decided who the headman should be, but now it is people from the town who establish the leader, as he has to speak Thai. The people from the village would choose someone who was a good hunter, a good fighter, and who was quite rich. The word of the headman is like a law; he is entitled to expel people from the village and even kill them if they do bad things like stealing or murder." Traditionally, the most common way of resolving conflict with the headman was for the affected families to go elsewhere and either set up their own village or move to another one. Households unwilling to conform to the leader moved away; those willing to conform stayed put.

As everyone in the village seemed to know that we were staying with the headman we were not besieged for money and sweets, although no one seemed to like having their photograph taken. This village had running water and the standpipes were obviously a great centre for social interaction at this time of the day, with people coming to wash, collect water or just have a chat. One of Emma's new friends took us to a small stream where a group of children were washing and playing around. The water was freezing but Emma seemed really to enjoy it, although her little friend seemed most upset that we didn't wash Emma's clothes. Trying to explain the difficulties of carrying around wet washing when we were moving on the next day was beyond my powers of communication when I didn't know a word of the language. As we walked back after the sun had set we saw the house of the resident schoolmistress shining out like a beacon. She was the only one in the village with an electric light, which was powered by a small solar panel.

As we sat in the house after our meal, a succession of people came and looked at us and seemed to be extremely interested in our books. Emma's books generated quite a lot of interest because of the pictures, but even Peter's large and boring paperback was looked at and the pages were turned over with wonderment. Several of the children wanted to carry it around but had to be restrained, as it was already starting to fall apart. My writing was another source of interest, and many people came to sit and watch me as I did this. The Lahu language has no traditional script, although Christian missionaries in Burma developed a Romanized written script. Outside China few Lahu other than Christians are literate in their own language. When we went to the school, such teaching materials as there were were all in Thai.

By the flickering light of the fire, in the room where everyone cooked, ate and slept, Nargat was very keen to talk about her experiences as a woman living in the village, and of pregnancy and birth. She spoke very easily to Dang without needing her husband either to translate or to give her moral support: "I've lived in three different places and this is the fourth place I've lived in. I think we've been here about nine years. When we were living in other places the trouble was that when we grew things the Thais who lived around in other villages would steal them. We don't really like living too close to the Thais, although those around here are very friendly and come to trade with us. We now understand that we mustn't cut down any trees, so we don't do it any more." She was very hazy about her age and couldn't remember how old she was when she got married: "The average age of getting married here is about sixteen but you can get married at any age after that. I think most women like to marry as soon as they can after they're sixteen and that's probably what I did. My husband came to live with my mother for about a year before we moved out to our own house."

In Lahu households relationships are traced through the female side, although the eldest man is usually the head.

When a man marries he goes to live with his wife's family and won't move out to build his own house until another sister gets married and brings in another son-in-law. The son-in-law has a very low status and is expected to do as he is told by the wife's father, although he will have his own hearth within the wife's house where his family will do their own cooking. Nargat had two fireplaces in her house, but only one was in use as none of her six children was yet old enough to be married. In this family, individuals owned only their personal clothes and maybe one or two other small items; the rest belonged to the household as a whole and could be used by any of them.

My inquiries about midwives and whether Nargat had ever had any help from one showed me once again just how misleading it can be to make assumptions about how other people live! Nargat was extremely surprised that I should think that most women needed outside help with giving birth: "Most Lahu girls know how to give birth by themselves, and they'll call the midwife only if it's very painful or if there's a lot of blood. When I was a little girl I watched the midwife deliver a lot of babies, so I knew what to do. My husband also watched the midwife when he was little, so he knew what to do as well; in fact he helped me when our second child was being born." Nargat delivered her first baby entirely on her own: "I was quite scared with the first pregnancy, but as the first birth was easy I wasn't scared any more. When I gave birth I squatted down and held on to the wall. [Lahu houses have convenient bars along the wall to which the split bamboo is tied, and these are just the right height for holding on to when squatting.] This is the best position, as it's easier to push; you can pull against the wall as you push. For me it has never been painful, although some women scream a lot." Nargat felt, however, that she was more stoical and perhaps more private than some of the other women in the village, and she didn't want anyone there apart from her husband: "My husband is the only person who has helped me in all my births; but that is fairly usual amongst us Lahu women. Other women in the village might ask for the midwife, but not my friends

32

and I – I think because we are strong. I'm scared that if the midwife came she might use her hands to help the baby out. I wouldn't like that, I'd be too embarrassed. I didn't even like my husband looking at me, so he helped me from behind." As Nargat explained, she was not used to anyone seeing her body: "Even when we have sex he doesn't see my body, as we do it in the dark."

After the baby was born Nargat cut the cord herself, tying it first with a piece of cotton before cutting it with a pair of scissors. Her husband put the placenta into a bamboo pipe and buried it, as was customary, under the hut. Then she did what all the other women did to recover from the birth: "I rested close to the fire for seven days or so and drank a lot of hot water, as I did all through the birth. My husband stayed close to me and used a hot towel to massage my stomach and get rid of all the bad blood." As there is no milk in the breasts immediately after birth, the baby is fed by another woman who already has milk; Nargat believed there was nothing of value in her breast until the milk came, and that if the baby needed anything this would have to be given by another breastfeeding mother. If the milk doesn't come, this is because of the interference of the spirits, and appropriate action has to be taken: "We kill a chicken and give it to the spirit and the milk always comes after a day or two." Babies are usually breastfed for about a year, after which they are taught to eat rice. Nargat stayed in the house for fifteen days, after which she went back to work in the rice fields, although this was fairly unusual: "I was able to take things easily while I was pregnant and after the birth, as my husband did all the work in the fields. After having the baby it's all right for the mother to go back to work in the rice fields after seven days, and lots of Lahu girls do. But my husband was very kind and said I could stay in the house a bit longer to make sure that I regained my strength properly." When she started work again she took the baby wrapped up in a towel. Babies who are still being breastfed are taken to the fields, but as they get older they tend to be looked after by their grandparents: "After my first baby was born there was a gap of about three and a half years before the next one came, and there's been that sort of gap between them all."

Nargat had several times referred to the spirits and how these might interfere and have to be dealt with during pregnancy and birth. The Lahu vary widely in their beliefs and practices, and have been influenced by other religions while not necessarily losing the basis of their own. They have a belief in a supreme deity which they call Ka-sa, but this deity is relatively removed from the good and bad spirits which are of far more consequence to humans and have to be propitiated. By far the most important spirit is the house spirit, as Nargat's husband explained: "Each house in a Lahu village has a spirit house which is a small room of bamboo in the main room of the house. I don't know the name of the spirit, but it is very powerful and can cause headaches and that sort of thing." In other places the house spirit is not thought to have any sort of evil intent, and in fact places a protective shield around the members of the household. Sometimes illness is thought to occur when the protective shield gets weak, perhaps because the house spirit has been offended or offerings have not been regularly made. In this village, however, the explanation seemed to be in terms of how far the house spirit could protect the household members when they went too far from the house: "The spirit in the house is like a sort of ancestor spirit and is very kind and good and looks after everyone who is in the house. People therefore get ill only if they go into the jungle, where the house spirit cannot protect them. Most people get ill because of fierce spirits in the jungle who attack them."

A person's physical body is thought to have a spiritual counterpart in the form of one or more souls. At death the soul goes to the land of the dead unless the person experienced a "bad death" – one involving violence – in which case he might return as a malicious spirit and cause a lot of ill fortune in the village. Otherwise the person will eventually be reborn as a human being. Illness is thought to be caused by the spirits attacking one or more of the souls, which then wander and cause the body to display symptoms of illness. In this case various rituals must be undertaken: "First of all I will kill a chicken or pig and leave it in the spirit room for the spirit. Then I make a bamboo platform and put some flowers on it. I then ask the spirit to take the illness out of the person and put it on the platform. I'll use my hands to help the spirit do this. We then take the platform out to the jungle and leave it there, and the illness will leave the person. It's like giving the illness back to the jungle spirit."

While all illness has a spiritual dimension, it is only the more serious illnesses that require these special rituals, as a less serious illness can be cured with medicine alone. Which spirit is causing the illness will be divined by the "spirit doctor", who will look at recent events, dreams, and so on to find out the cause. It is up to him to decide which is the most appropriate ritual and how many of the family or the villagers need to be involved, although as the headman said, this might require a certain amount of trial and error: "If you are ill you take medicine, but it doesn't always work first time and if it doesn't then you try something else. It's exactly the same with different rituals – if one doesn't work, we try something else." Sometimes, of course, one just has to bow to the inevitable: "If we try everything and you don't get any better, then we just have to leave it. In that case the spirit has decided that you should be ill and there's nothing we can do about it."

We were staying in the village during the cold season, when many people caught colds and flu. While there are few rituals to prevent illness, that night there was going to be a special celebration which it was hoped would protect the village from too much disease: "Tonight we are going to sacrifice a pig and dance to the spirit in the hope that it won't cause any problems. Someone from every family in the village will do this." Later I found out that the dancing had been organized by the family of a woman suffering from stomach problems. The mother had killed a pig, which she had shared, and was expecting that the dancing would also help cure the sickness. Other families were hoping that by participating they would obtain more general protection. We went to the dancing with the headman's son, who took with him a wind instrument with which he was going to play to the spirits. This gave out a breathy sound, rather like bagpipes without enough puff. The dancing was being held in a special area which had been fenced off and consisted of a dancing circle of beaten earth in the middle of which was a mound. On the mound were some candles whose small flickering light was all there was to see by as the men and women danced around in pairs of the same sex. To the sound of a banjo-like instrument and several wind instruments, fifteen or sixteen people danced around to the regular beat of the men's stamping feet. When this was done in unison it had quite a hypnotic effect although the women did their own, much more delicate, footwork.

This went on for some time, but it was cold if you weren't a dancer and we were glad to go back to the warmth of the house and sleep round the fire. Nargat's children decided they wanted to sleep in our car, which must have been freezing, although in the morning they assured us that they had had a wonderful night!

Before leaving the next morning we were able to talk to Nami, the headman's sister, who apparently had a very good reputation for being able to help people who were ill as well as mothers with pregnancy and birth. Every year she helped with three or four births, sometimes in villages that were as far as a two-day trek away. Despite the general feeling that she was particularly gifted for this work, she hadn't received any special tuition or knowledge: "Nobody taught me how to be a midwife, although I used to watch the midwife working when I was young. In my heart I knew that I wanted to help people, especially after watching a baby being born." She began practising after giving birth to her first two children: "I gave birth to my children on my own and . . . I don't know . . . people used to say that as I'd given birth on my own, I'd be able to help others. They started coming to me for my help and I suppose I've been doing it for about twenty-five years now."

Most women didn't see Nami during their pregnancy unless

there was something amiss: "Mostly women don't come to me until the baby is ready to be born. If they need help

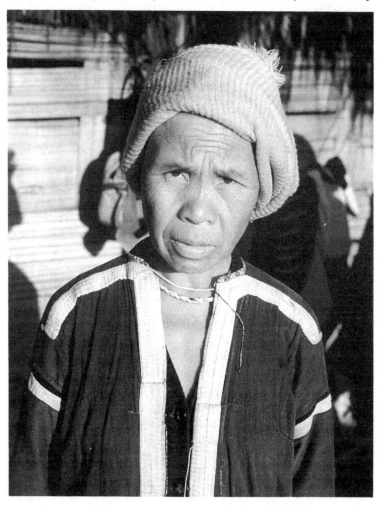

Nami, the midwife in the Black Lahu village

before that – perhaps because they have pains in their belly, or something like that – then their husband will come to get me. Sometimes if the baby is lying in the wrong position it can be very painful, and backache is sometimes another problem. Headache and dizziness can also be experienced, especially in the beginning. For the backache and stomach pains I give massage, but if she is dizzy and vomiting – well! That's just nature's way.

"When a woman is ready to give birth, her husband will come and get me. The first thing I do is to touch her stomach so that I can tell when the baby is going to be born. I massage her and wait for the white liquid to come out, and this can take up to three days. I stay with her the whole time, give her massage, encourage her to take hot water and say good things to her to help her through the pains. Anyone can come and visit, and the women especially usually do. We all sit around and drink tea and try to console her. Sometimes the baby and everything comes out very quickly, but sometimes the baby comes out and the placenta comes out an hour or two later. I can't cut the cord until the placenta comes out, nor feed or bath the baby. While we're waiting I'll massage the mother. Once the placenta comes I can cut the cord, which I do with bamboo or scissors. Yes, we bury the placenta under the house. It is an agreement with our spirits, and if we don't the baby could become ill."

Like Nargat, Nami was very definite about the best way of giving birth: "Squatting and holding on to the wall is the best position for giving birth. I stand behind the woman and I massage her until the baby comes out." After the birth the mother will be massaged by the husband, using a warm towel, and the baby will not be bathed for up to fifteen days. Nami said that she would call in to see the mother three or four times during the next seven to fifteen days to see that everything was all right. Payment depended on the means of the family, and could be in kind: "Ten years ago I would be paid by either the woman's husband or other male relative coming to help me in the rice field. But now money is important and they will pay me B50 or B100, but if they can't afford it one of the family will come and help in the rice fields."

For any minor problems of pregnancy Nami said that she would kill a chicken and leave it with some whisky in the spirit room. If there was excessive pain during the birth she would massage to help the baby move and to take the soreness away.

She showed me how she did this: I sat down cross-legged and she sat down behind me. She started by massaging around my stomach, pushing her fingers in quite deeply and systematically all the way round: "I can tell whether a baby is there, even quite early on. If the baby is in the wrong position, which is painful for the mother, I can move it, but I don't try and turn a breech baby round. Did you know that boys tend to lie on the right-hand side and girls on the left?" If a woman had pains in the top of her belly, Nami showed me how she pulled her back so she was arched over her knee, then she would massage around her belly. When she did this to me it felt much more comfortable than the explanation might suggest.

One of the most surprising things to me was Nami's categorical denial of ever having to deal with a perineal tear: "We Lahu women don't tear when we give birth." I asked Dang to explain again precisely what I meant, and to tell her that where I come from this is very common. But she was quite adamant: "No, never in all my experience have I seen a woman tear there and no, I don't have to use oil or do anything else to stop the tearing. The babies just come out naturally in their own time." Although she had mentioned waiting for the placenta to come out, she said she had never had to wait more than an hour so she didn't see it as a problem. She had experienced a breech birth but said that this was very rare: "Babies nearly always come out head first but sometimes they come out feet first, and it's much more painful. I know another midwife who is able to put her hand inside and make the baby do a somersault so it comes out head first. But I don't do this, I just let the baby come out feet first."

On the whole mothers did not have problems with breastfeeding and, like Nargat, Nami thought that provided a chicken was killed there should be no problems. On the rare occasions when the milk either didn't come or was insufficient, Nami advised the woman to find a special herb which grew deep in the jungle. Generally there were no food restrictions after giving birth, although Nami said that some mothers didn't eat garlic, salty fish or pickles as it made them feel ill.

The Lahu have no traditional forms of contraception: "If we don't want to have any more babies we have to stop sleeping together." Nargat said that although other people had more children, after six she had had enough: "Lahu people believe that it is good to have a lot of children, maybe ten or twelve, but six is enough for me!" Her husband added: "The more children you have the better and we believe, even now, that children help to increase your production and show how strong your wife is. Every year in the past two or three babies would die, but now fewer do so and last year no babies in this village died. I think it's because people are more careful about what they eat and drink and we don't have to work as hard as we did. The government also teaches us about sanitation and will give us medicine if we need it." Despite being so close to the road and "civilization", no one seemed to know about modern methods of contraception.

The next Lahu village, one belonging to the so-called Red Lahu, was as far from the road as the other one was near. It took an hour or so to walk there along open paths with nothing to shield us from the hot sun. All around were denuded hills, some with one or two straggling trees standing in splendid but sorrowful isolation. It was difficult to imagine these hills being covered with trees, as they must once have been and in some cases will be again, although in future they will be covered in pine trees planted in rows rather than luxuriant jungle.

The village was in a valley surrounded by hills and consisted of a lower village (where we stayed) and a higher part which was reached by climbing up a very steep slope. At the top of this slope was a huge house which, because of its size and the fact that it was made out of planks rather than bamboo, seemed to dominate this part of the village. This house also sported a television aerial, although I never discovered where they plugged it in as the village had no electricity. I was exhorted by several of the villagers to try the shower, which was in a small room at the end of this house, and of which they were obviously very proud. The pipe for the water went vertically up the slope, ending at the shower head, which was stuck at a crazy angle in the wall of the room, dripping furiously and keeping everything very wet and slippery. Although it was at the top of the hill the water gushed out very fast – so fast, in fact, that as Dang said, you didn't notice how cold it was. The house where we stayed was much less grand, being made of bamboo and consisting of one large room where all family activities took place. I slept in a special little guest room which had been built on at the front, as this was one of the villages where trekkers often spent the night.

The husband (Jeti) and wife (Naby) who owned the house were both opium smokers and smiled up at us cheerily through a haze of smoke as they reclined on the floor, puffing happily. The whole village had a very relaxed and laid-back feeling about it, partly because this was a time of the year when hard work such as planting or harvesting was not necessary, so everyone could have a rest. Despite my rather censorious feelings about people who lie around all day taking drugs, I couldn't help liking this couple, who didn't seem so far gone that they were neglecting either their family or themselves. They were very happy to talk, and I spent most of the day sitting around with them discussing village life, love and birth. Jeti told me about his courtship of Naby: "Everyone in this village used to live about seventy-five kilometres away, and then fifteen years ago everyone moved here. We knew each other as neighbours in the other place, but by the time we came here our love was growing and eventually we got married." Jeti then explained in great and energetic detail the courting customs of the village, which seemed very relaxed: "Young people like to prove they're growing up by sleeping together. Every evening the young men and the women go out looking for each other, and then they pair off into the jungle and make love."

I had some evidence of this on the night I stayed there. As well as the young driver's son we had also brought with us a young man from another village. Throughout the evening a succession of nubile young women called at the house to say hello and to try and engage the young men in conversation. Unfortunately I was too tired to stay up and see if this came to anything or not, and everyone kept their mouths very firmly closed when I asked about it the next morning. Jeti, who liked to think of himself as something of a rake, merely remarked, "The boys like to try out all the girls, and when I was young I'd fucked the whole village!"

Despite this seemingly relaxed attitude towards sex, virginity was prized, and the fact that Naby was a virgin when she got married made her quite a catch. Jeti thought that by marrying her he had got the best of both worlds: "Naby was very skinny and rather sickly when she was young and so she didn't participate in all this running around. If she wasn't beautiful that was all the better for me, because I was her first." There can be problems if a woman has an illegitimate baby, and it is not unknown for women to be expelled from the village if they become pregnant and don't manage to find themselves a husband.

Once a couple are married, the women seem to take the upper hand in deciding whether to stay married or not, as Jeti was well aware: "If, after you get married, you find you don't like the man or you don't have any children, then you can separate easily. I know one woman who was married to six different men; they all turned out to be addicts and they didn't help her in the fields, so she got rid of them. The man has to be a good husband and help his wife in their fields, otherwise she gets rid of him." Once married the man went to live with the woman's family for a time before setting up their own house. Jeti, however, had liked his in-laws and had stayed with them until they died. Their first baby had died after a few months and about eighteen months after that Naby had given birth to twin boys, who were both very healthy. This had been quite a shock, given that Naby was not considered to be the strongest of women. I don't know whether Jeti and Naby were using contraception to limit their family, which was extremely small by village standards.

"In the past, women would have as many babies as they could, maybe twelve or thirteen, until their wombs didn't work any more. Nowadays we get pills from the lady by the waterfall and she explains how to take them. The right number of children to have now is two or three" (said Jeti).

"No! That's not right – it's four or five" (said Naby).

But they both agreed that in the past most people had too many children.

Knowing that I was interested in talking to a midwife they introduced me to Larni, an older woman, probably about sixty-five, who helped many of the village women with pregnancy and birth: "I'm just one of a number of older women who are asked to help if there are women who feel they need it. Mostly a woman will be helped by her friends. Most women know what to do; it's something a mother teaches her daughter when she is young. All the women and men in this village know a lot about giving birth; they can do the massage as well as me." Like many older women Larni was a widow, her husband having died of opium addiction. She was married when she was about fifteen and had eight children altogether, although three of them had died, she thought from stomach problems, mainly diarrhoea.

If Larni's help was required, it was usually requested once the woman had gone into labour: "I help a woman in labour by sitting behind her with my knees in her back and massaging her belly." At the same time her friends would all be around her helping: "Her friends would help by telling dirty jokes." What sort of dirty jokes? "Oh! You know, talking about what goes in before the baby comes out, and all that sort of thing. It helps to keep her spirits up." In Larni's experience it was usually only a few hours before the baby came out: "To give birth the woman kneels down and holds on to a stick or something above her head, then I will squat with her with my knees in her back and if necessary I will massage her stomach to help the baby come out." If it looks as if it will take a long time, the magic man is summoned and various rituals are undertaken to pacify the house spirit and other spirits that might be causing the problems.

As in the previous village, the cord was not cut until the placenta was delivered, Larni tying the cord with cotton about an inch from the belly before cutting it with a piece of bamboo. The mother would then lie by the fire with the baby for twelve days or so, the husband massaging her stomach with a hot towel to expel all the blood. Larni bathed the baby after birth, but the mother was not allowed to bathe for at least two days afterwards: "Then the husband has to find a mother who is feeding a baby so that she can feed his newborn baby until the milk comes after a couple of days." Larni had never experienced breastfeeding problems: "The milk always comes and there's no need to do anything like taking special herbs to make it come." There were no real dietary restrictions, although chicken was thought to be a good food to eat after birth: "The mother eats only chicken and rice for the first twelve to fifteen days. Sometimes a family has to kill more than twenty chickens at this time. Eating chicken helps to expel the bad blood, and in that way it is just like a herb. After six weeks the mother will start working in the fields again."

Also as in the other village, there were no rituals connected with pregnancy or birth, and the naming was an informal affair decided by the parents. The name could mean anything; Jeti, for instance, said that his name meant "born in the morning". For the Lahu in both villages birth continues to be a family event: a normal part of family life, with most of the necessary help coming from relatives and only in very exceptional cases from outsiders.

4

ARE THE SPIRITS HAPPY?: BIRTH AMONGST THE AKKHA

THE PATH UP TO the Akkha village of Banhuang was steep and twisting and as I struggled up, leaning forward to counteract the weight of my rucksack, I felt that at times my nose must touch the path. Focusing my whole concentration on putting one foot in front of the other and heaving myself up the next step, I thought what a perfect demonstration it was of how the Akkha like to live in the more inaccessible parts of northern Thailand, with their villages on or near the tops of the higher slopes. As we got nearer the top, some boys from the village swooped down on us with delighted cries. Dang was well known and liked in this village and regularly brought groups of visitors, so his arrival was always a cause for celebration. The boys took some of our bags and ran back up the path to tell everyone else about our arrival, their speed and surefootedness putting my plodding, gasping progress to shame.

The first thing we saw of the village was the spirit gate, which stretched across the path up which we had just climbed. This was a fairly rough structure composed of two upright bamboo poles, with a large pole across the top. It was decorated with all manner of abstract constructions, with carvings of birds and animals. In other villages I also saw carvings of more modern items like aeroplanes and helicopters. At the foot of the gate were two carved wooden figures with exaggerated genitals. These symbolized man and woman, rejuvenating the fertility of everyone in the village and ensuring the everlasting reproduction of the Akkha race. The object of the spirit gate is to prevent all the bad spirits which live in the jungle from coming into the village. The gate is renewed each year, and as the year progresses its power gradually lessens. Just before a new gate is erected all the bad spirits which have managed to slip through into the village in the previous year are driven out by the young boys using sticks. There is a gate on the main path which enters at each end of the village; they protect not only this path but all that is within the boundary of the village.

As we walked into the village we were met by some of the younger women, who were dressed in short black mini-skirts and leggings. Most of them also wore black tops, although a few of them continued to go topless in the traditional way. At least no one was wearing a bra as a top, which I think looks most peculiar with this traditional dress. I always think it is a pity that, having in the past persuaded groups such as these to become conscious and ashamed of not covering their breasts, we now proceed to shock them by doing just that ourselves. The most distinctive feature of women's dress was their beautifully decorated hats. For everyday wear the hat consisted of a simple beaded length of material which fitted round the head like a large skullcap. It had all manner of decorations hanging down from it, including lengths of beads and dyed chicken feathers with, across the forehead, a string of Indian coins. Young girls wear a simple cloth cap and as they grow older add bead and feather decorations and, when they attain puberty, the string of Indian rupees across their foreheads. In this village unmarried women wore the hat well down over their forehead so that the hairline didn't show, but once they were married they wore it further back to show their hair, which was kept in place by a series of long hairpins. Women are very attached to their hats and, so I was told, rarely take them off, not even to go to bed!

We walked through the village past the so-called "courting

place", a flat cleared area with benches around it. Much has been made of this in the literature as a place where the young people gather in the evening to sing, flirt, and decide with whom they would like to have sex. Unfortunately I never saw it being used, maybe because we were a greater source of entertainment and they preferred to come and look at us instead. Or maybe everyone was just working too hard and didn't have to time and energy for these activities. This village was quite small, with only a dozen houses set in two parallel lines along the saddle of the hill. Walking through, I realized just how high up we were, especially at night when it was possible to see the lights of the town twinkling away in the far distance. The Akkha like to have a ring of trees around the village from which they gather their firewood and maybe some wild fruits, but with the lack of land this is getting more difficult to arrange and most villages are not surrounded by trees as this one was. Most villages are quite small but there are some with up to 200 houses, although these are unusual as the Akkha much prefer to live in small remote settlements where they won't be disturbed. Of all the hill tribes the Akkha have been the least willing to communicate with outsiders, preferring to continue with their way of life on their own.

As they prefer their villages to be so high, many Akkha build on watersheds where there is no natural source of water. Usually they carry water to their houses from the lower slopes, and I saw how this job takes up a lot of the time of the younger women and children. There is a saying amongst the hill tribes that "Water flows to all the hill tribes except the Akkha, who have to fetch their own." Later that evening, after we had settled in, I went down to the water place and found this out for myself. I slithered down a steep, muddy path to where the water had been diverted with a bamboo pipe from a small stream to form a continuous shower. Here we waited in turn as women filled up their water containers, which included plastic bottles as well as traditional bamboo water pipes and gourds. Many of them brought their water containers down in baskets, and I helped one little girl to put the basket of full containers on her back before carrying it up to the village. I could hardly lift it and couldn't imagine how she was going to carry it up the steep slithery slope, but she went off at a steady trot, not slowing down as she toiled upwards. As we waited our turn for the water we saw the women coming in from the fields carrying large bundles of thatching material. These bundles were about the same diameter as their bodies and about twice as tall as themselves, and as they walked, or rather trotted, down the steep winding paths they looked in imminent danger of overbalancing, although as far as we knew no one ever did. Coming to the water, they would stop to wash before taking up their bundles once again and walking up to the village. At that time of the evening the water place was obviously a favourite meeting spot, with everyone exchanging gossip and a lot of good-natured laughing and bantering between the young men and women.

In this village we stayed at a special "guesthouse" which had been built, at Dang's instigation and with his financial help, by Amon, one of the villagers. Amon was an opium addict and smoked continuously both day and night with a desperation and intensity that I hadn't seen in the other villages where smoking seemed to be much more of a social lubricant, rather like alcohol or marijuana. Here there were few men in evidence going about the village, and according to Dang this was because most of them smoked opium. Much to my delight, Amon's wife Ammer had given birth to a little boy three weeks earlier. I was captivated by him and stroked his forehead. Unfortunately Dang had forgotten to tell me that I shouldn't touch him, as even though the people of this village are used to strangers, there is an ingrained feeling that anyone coming from outside may bring with them evil spirits. Fortunately there was a way to overcome my gaffe and to neutralize any possible evil influences that I may inadvertently have brought with me. I tied a piece of cotton round the baby's wrist and put some silver in his hand to show that my intentions were good. After this I sat down to give Emma a suck, whereupon the new baby's smallest sister came and seemed to be very interested in what was going on. Later I found out that since the baby had arrived she had not been allowed to suck any more. As a consequence she was very vulnerable and rather insecure, and when Emma ran off to play she immediately placed herself on my lap for a cuddle.

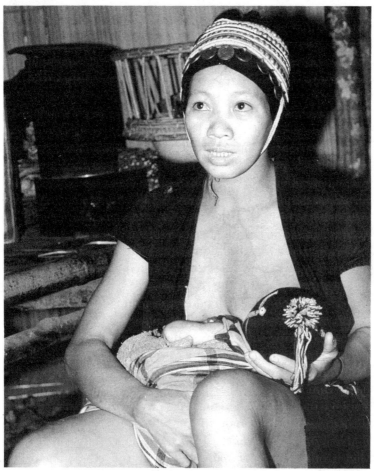

Ammer nursing her three week old baby

All over the village, on roofs and on the ground, bundles of grass for making the local brooms (which are used by everyone in Thailand) were lying out to dry. Later we all helped Ammer's eldest daughter to strip off the seeds and the smaller twigs before they were laid out to dry again and then sold in the town. The Akkha economy is very self-contained and they are able to grow most of the crops they need for survival. Like other hill tribes it is based on swidden agriculture, although with the lack of land and where the terrain is suitable (which is not all that often in these higher hills) some are turning to the more sustainable terracing of the land and wet rice cultivation. Rice is their chief crop, although they also grow a very wide range of vegetables, cotton and tobacco. Opium is the chief cash crop and they also breed pigs, oxen, goats and chickens, some of which they sell. They are also supposed particularly to enjoy eating dog meat, and much of what I have read suggests that dog meat is as important to the Akkha as pork is to other groups, but I didn't see any evidence of this. They are also said to be expert hunters, although they don't have much opportunity now in the depleted forests. Apparently, when Amon had sowed the rice in the previous year he had mixed up all the different seeds so that the harvest was a curious mixture of the chewy hill rice together with sticky glutinous rice. Here, of course, there was no question of overcoming the mistake by buying all the rice for the next year, as this would have been prohibitively expensive. There was nothing for it, but to eat it all up and make sure that the same mistake wasn't made next year. I think it affected us much less than Dang, who like most locals was quite a connoisseur of rice and found the mixture most unpalatable.

Like many of the northern hill tribes in Thailand, the Akkha come from the southern provinces of China. They migrated from Yunnan to the Burmese Shan states and from there to northern Thailand about sixty or seventy years ago. They are the smallest of the ethnic minorities of Thailand, numbering around 10,000, although they are far more numerous in China and Burma. In Thailand most of the Akkha live in the northern Chiang Rai province. They speak a Tibeto-Burman language which is closely related to Lahu and Lisu (other ethnic groups amongst the hill tribes) but do not have a written language. According to one legend they used to have their own alphabet, which was inscribed on a buffalo hide, but this was stolen and eaten by a dog, and since then there has been no written language. They are probably the poorest and least developed ethnic minority in Thailand, with a low standard of living which stems in part from the inaccessible places in which they prefer to live and their desire to continue living in their own self-sufficient way without the intervention of strangers.

The "guesthouse" in which we stayed was built along the same lines as a traditional Akkha house with uprights of bamboo, walls of split bamboo and a thatched roof. On each side of the long hut were sleeping platforms, and – luxury for this sort of accommodation – proper mattresses. Apparently Dang had persuaded Amon to buy these, and had even lent him the money to do so, as he said that more visitors would thereby be encouraged to come. We visited Amon's house often, as the entrance to it was opposite the entrance to the guesthouse and all the cooking was done in his home. Like all Akkha houses it had a steep pitched roof which sloped in four (instead of the usual two) directions almost to the floor. It was not built on stilts but inside, on the left, was a sleeping platform where Amon lay for most of the night and day, puffing at his opium pipe. At one end of the house, on the floor, was the cooking fire, which burned continuously, the smoke curling up to the roof and seeping out of the windowless house through the thatch and the split bamboo walls.

I don't know whether Amon's house was particularly simple or whether I was just unaware of some of the refinements which have been seen by other visitors to these villages. As many Akkha houses are built on a slope they often stand completely on piles, so that the floor can be levelled, although most contain a higher sleeping platform at one side. What is most characteristic, however, is the way in which the house is divided into a women's and a men's section. Amon did refer to this with regard to the sleeping arrangements, but apart from this men and women seemed to mix in the house, although this may have been because we were guests and the strictures therefore didn't apply to the same degree. There is an ancestral altar (in Amon's case it was very simple and I wouldn't have noticed it if he hadn't pointed it out to me), and it is this which usually divides the house up between the women's and men's section. Sometimes each side of the house has its own fireplace, or there is one fireplace at the boundary of the two sections. Rice is prepared on the women's side, while tea and other things are prepared on the men's side, but in Amon's house everything appeared to be cooked on the one fire. Outside the door leading from the women's section of the house is the rice pounder and outside the men's section is an open platform which is used for a wide range of activities, from washing up and drying vegetables to sitting on in the evening.

The next morning we sat on the sleeping platform and talked to Ammer and Amon. I had met Ammer the previous year when she had been the driving force behind looking after the visitors and obviously ran all the household activities. Not surprisingly, this time she was very centred on the baby, and although she did join in the conversation from time to time she spent most of the time doing things for him, occasionally stopping for a few easy household tasks. Amon, despite smoking opium in his usual intense way, was remarkably lucid and tended to dominate the conversation. I would have liked to speak more to Ammer, but since she was so focused on the baby and showed a natural inclination to let her husband take the lead, this wasn't possible. In this village women were expected to do most of the work and submit to their husbands' wishes. I was surprised that her husband's opium smoking was so acceptable to Ammer; in fact it seemed to be all part of a macho image that showed her husband was a "real man" – he could take his opium and he was a good hunter, and this made him very desirable. Whether this was just her own rationalization or an opinion shared by all the other women in the village I never found out. The Akkha women certainly seemed very strong and forthright, and I was surprised they put up with such behaviour from their men, but I was assured by both Ammer and Amon that this was how things were.

Ammer told us about her marriage: "I got married when I

was seventeen and he was eighteen which was quite young compared to other people. In the past people got married when they were about twenty-three years old, but any time after the age of fifteen is all right. The most important thing is that the couple are happy together." There has been endless discussion in the literature about the sexual licence enjoyed by young Akkha people, and according to Amon and Ammer this was true for them – but with, it seemed to me, many more advantages for the man than the woman. If a woman becomes pregnant, she has to name the father of the baby, but if he denies it and won't marry her, the woman becomes an evil omen and is expelled from the village until her child is born, when she can return but must build a new house for herself. Fortunately for Ammer, Amon didn't reject her: "When the woman gets married she has to go and live with her husband's family and they live all together until they need more room, when the young couple move out and build their own place." This will to some extent depend on how many sons the family has as one of them, with his wife and children, must continue to live with the parents to care for them in their old age: "I lived with my husband's family for a year, but none of us was very happy. My father-in-law was a very bad-tempered man and horrible to us, so we decided to move out and build our own house." Amon's father was in fact the headman of the village, and as the eldest son Amon could have expected to take over this role when his father died. When he grew up and became addicted to opium, the resulting conflict between him and his father led to his giving up the idea of becoming headman. Amon's brother took up the post instead and, although somewhat young for the position, had the necessary industry and financial backing, with the added advantage of speaking Thai.

Children are thought to belong to the father's ancestors as the wife is considered to belong to the husband's family. Although in theory it is possible for an Akkha man to have three wives, in practice he is unlikely to have more than one unless she is infertile. In theory again, divorce is simple, especially if there are no children, when fines will be paid as laid down by the headman. A divorced wife cannot go back to her parents, however, and must either remarry within twelve days or live outside the village. Perhaps most divorces come about as a result of adultery, which can then be transformed into another marriage once the divorce is through.

Ammer spoke with some bitterness about the birth and subsequent death of her first baby, which she felt had been brought about by her in-laws: "I became pregnant after we'd been married about a year and had a little boy, but when he was six months old he died. I don't know why, but right from the beginning he was always weak and coughed a lot. We didn't have any money so we couldn't take him to the hospital and my father-in-law wouldn't give us any money to do so. If he had lived he would be about fourteen years old now. I had to work very hard indeed in that house, and yet when the baby was ill they wouldn't give us any money to take him to hospital. Afterwards we moved right away from the village, but in the end we came back." As Ammer explained, it was very important for an Akkha family to have at least one son, so she was very upset by her first baby's death: "The Akkha way is to make sure that you always have at least one son, and if you don't have any then your husband is entitled to get another wife. This is because when girls marry they have to move to their husband's family, and if you have all girls there will be no one to look after you when you are old. When girls marry they may charge the man's family two or three pigs or something like that as compensation, although it's much more nowadays."

During pregnancy both husband and wife observe certain restrictions to ensure that their baby will not be either deformed or twins, both of which are rejected in Akkha society. They avoid all spiritually powerful people such as priests and shamans and don't participate in religious activities, burial parties or hunting expeditions, all of which can lead to confrontation with evil spirits. For Ammer, however, the main preoccupation was whether she would have a boy after previously giving birth to three girls: "I was scared of having another daughter, as after having three girls we desperately wanted another boy. We had a lot of arguments, as he said that if I had another girl he would marry someone else. If he couldn't father a boy, people in the village would ask: 'Why can't she give you a son? You have been a good husband and it would be better if you took a new wife.' Then he would say to me that our love was over and that he was going to take a new wife. We asked the spirits for a son and cut all the girls' hair off so that it was short like a boy's. We thought it would help us to have a son, and it did." With only one son, however, Ammer was still aware of the precariousness of her position: "I think having four or five children is about right, but my neighbours say that I ought to have another son in case this one dies." There is no traditional method of birth control, and in fact large numbers of children are still liked: "In the past we tried to have as many children as possible. My husband's mother had eleven, but five of them died. You need lots of children so that you have plenty of help in the rice fields, and of course it also increases the size of the community."

Ammer then went on to tell me about her labour and birth: "While a woman is in labour she must not drink cold water, only hot. We use only one herb for pregnancy and birth, which we call Shigo [the Thais call it Red Bhanken]. We boil this with hot water and then drink the liquid to expel all the dried-up blood that's left inside after giving birth." Akkha midwives are older women and preferably those who have given birth to several sons, although they are used only by women with no family nearby. This was the case for Ammer: "When the pains came, Amon went to get the midwife. Once he has gone to get her he mustn't come inside the house again until the baby is born. I don't know why that is so but if the husband was around in the house then the birth would be very difficult indeed – in fact she could find it impossible." Once the baby is born, it will not be picked up until it has cried, "begging God for a blessing, a soul and a lifespan". The midwife has to give the baby a name, which prevents the spirits naming and therefore taking it. This is not as difficult as it may seem, as Amon said: "We count from the first onwards, calling the first one 'first child' and so on, so she'll know what name to give it."

The cord is cut with a piece of bamboo and the husband is then allowed to enter the house, after which there are various rituals which both the man and the woman must undertake to ensure that the spirits are propitiated: "After I'd given birth, Amon boiled a chicken's egg and gave half to me and the other half to the baby. After that I was able to give the baby his first milk. Amon then killed a female chicken and cooked it. Some of the meat was given to me and some to the baby, after which he did the ceremony with the placenta."

Amon continued: "I mixed the chicken soup with the cord and the placenta and took it out to the house pole [this is a pole just outside the house to which the ancestors are thought to be attached]. I dug a hole and buried the placenta and put a stick over the place. Then every morning for seven days after that I poured boiling water over it and then I threw the stick away on to the land. In this way we make sure the cord will drop off the baby as fast as possible. After the birth of a baby we have to stay in the village for two days; we mustn't go outside into the jungle."

There were various taboos which Ammer also had to observe: "After giving birth I mustn't eat any blind animals, as the baby can't see properly for two months and if I ate anything like this he could stay permanently blind. Also I mustn't eat food that is too spicy, or sour fruit." Ammer was not allowed to leave the house for several days and there were various rituals related to this: "The day after the baby was born, Amon went out and found a pole which he put in the ground about fifteen metres from the house. He then took my wood basket and tied it on to the pole. After he'd put three sticks in the basket he came back and told me it was all right to go out now. I then took some water from the house, went to the pole and washed off all the blood and stuff left over from the delivery. Some of the water is used to wash the sticks, which are then brought back and burnt on the house fire. I don't know why we do this, it is just our Akkha way."

After birth the baby will be fed by another breastfeeding

56

woman until the milk comes after about three days, although Ammer did not find it necessary this time: "I already had milk, so there was food for the baby. Sometimes the woman has milk but the baby can't suck it out; then the husband has to suck first so that the baby can do it." If the family were poor the woman would probably go back to work in the fields after ten days or so, but this all depended on her husband and some women were able to rest for as long as two months. Ammer was not taking any chances: "I want to stay with my son for as long as possible to make sure that he is all right." Both of them thought that everyone was healthier now, as Amon put it: "In the past many babies and children died, but not now because we are more civilized. There are programmes on the radio in the Akkha language which teach us about drinking hot water and that sort of thing. We also trek to the town to the doctor if we need to. Every year we spend a lot of money at the hospital and sometimes I have to stop smoking for a week so that we can take the children there." It is a considerable trek along paths to a road, where the few public transport vans will not always pick up Akkha clients as they think this puts off other potential passengers.

During Ammer and Amon's description of birth and the rituals that surround it I was surprised at both their number and the particularity with which they were carried out. The most important justification for this seem to be that it was "the Akkha way", with no further explanation or justification being required to ensure that they were carried out as meticulously as possible. Compared to other hill tribe groups, the Akkha have a very large number of rituals which they continue to observe and with which they have a somewhat rueful relationship. Rituals are seen as a burden but also as a blessing, which is what makes the Akkha distinctive from any other group. The story they tell about this explains why they have so many and why they must continue to observe them: "Long ago the northern Thai, Chinese, Lahu, Lisu and Akkha people were given customs by the Creator. All the groups except the Akkha went to see the Creator with loosely woven baskets with wide spaces between the bamboo strips.

Some were also broken and torn. The Akkha, however, went to fetch the customs carrying the tightly woven basket used for carrying rice from the fields. Everyone put the customs in their baskets, but on the way home many of them fell through the gaps in the baskets and were lost. Because the Akkha put their customs in such a well-made, basket none of them was lost on the way back. That is why the customs of the Akkha are many whilst those of the other groups are few." Often the Akkha say "our customs are many and difficult", an observation which is made both proudly and deprecatingly. To complain that their customs are vast and demanding accounts for their lowly position *vis-à-vis* others, but at the same time praises the richness of the ancestors' bequest and the pride the Akkha feel in celebrating their own loyalty to that legacy.

The Akkha supernaturals include a supreme deity called A Po Mi Yeh, together with spirits and ancestors to whom offerings are made. The "Great spirits" include the sun and moon, who cannot harm but can be encouraged to help if properly propitiated. There are also "Owner spirits" in charge of livestock and the *padi*, who can be prayed to for help. These benign spirits live within the confines of the village; those less benign live outside. These include "Afflicting spirits" who can cause illness if offended, and spirits who enter people and can cause death unless they are driven out. At birth, marriage and death various rituals are performed to both the ancestors and spirits so that bad things are avoided. Regular village festivals also propitiate the spirits, and if the village as a whole is struck by disaster there are special rituals which can be enacted to neutralize this. Only if customs are carried out will blessings be received in the form of healthy children, animals and sufficient crops. It is possible, even then, that the ancestors and spirits may withhold their blessings, but if the customs are not followed they most certainly will.

Everyone has a soul which lives in the body, but it can and will leave if it gets frightened and if it cannot be brought back, the person will die. Before a child is weaned it is under the care of the spirit which causes pregnancy, and its welfare is thought to be bound up inextricably with that of the mother. After weaning it comes under the protection of the ancestors. Like human beings and unlike all other crops, rice is thought to have a soul and it is therefore used in rituals to provide a path to the ancestors, who will then protect the family against the spirits of the forest. Within the village there are a number of sacred places, one of which is the swing used in the New Year festival. Each village has two giant swings which are rebuilt every year for an annual four-day ceremony when everyone swings on them to celebrate the maturation of the rice and to thank the ancestors. Another very important place is the so-called "Creator's Water Source". This is usually located above the place from which the water is drawn for the village, and water will be drawn from it only for religious purposes such as when the village priest uses it for purifying the rice seeds used for the first planting.

The most important ritual specialist is the village priest; he is the first to take a bite at ceremonial meals, the first to have his house built in a new village, the first to plant *padi*, the instigator for building the spirit gates and swings and the first to start the New Year gambling. I couldn't make out whether Amon's father had been the village priest as well as the headman, as according to Amon he used to be responsible for instigating various village rituals to do with the supernatural. There are also "spirit priests" or shamans, normally women, who are able to communicate with the spirits and retrieve wandering spirits by going back to the land of ancestors. Each person is said to have a tree of life in this spirit world, and another task of the shaman is to visit the spirit world to see how this tree is getting on.

The "spirit doctor" for this village lived at another village nearby and was obviously held in high esteem by everyone. Although some villagers did use the hospital, the first recourse was always to the spirit doctor: "If we break something we always prefer to go to the magic man. We don't go to the doctor, as he will only cut you open and it is not necessary. I know someone who crushed his leg and the bones were all broken into little pieces, but this man managed to mend it.

We have our own herbs for every disease and we also have our own experts in magic." Some people had special gifts for curing – as Ammer described her father: "He was very good at healing badly cut fingers, even those which had been cut off. I have seen him take the herbs, say some magic and put the finger back on. I have seen him do this not once but four times."

Amon had promised that he would introduce me to the midwife and eventually, one evening when we were all sitting around surrounded by a cloud of wood and opium smoke, Atok, a small wizened woman of sixty, and Midok, a robust woman of about forty-five turned up. I had already met Midok, who had carried a rather weak and ill Emma about two miles over steep paths back to the village on one of the previous days. Like the midwives of the Lahu, they didn't think they had any special knowledge: "Midwifery is part of our Akkha way and everyone knows how to do it. Mothers teach their daughters how to deliver babies and when your daughter gets pregnant then the mother or the mother-in-law is the midwife. People come for me only if they don't have a mother or mother-in-law to help them." This, of course, had been true for Ammer, who was living in the village of her husband's family and whose in-laws were dead. Both Amok and Midok said that they had been taught by their mothers: "My mother said to me, 'I will teach you how to be a midwife and then you must teach your daughters and daughter-in-law so that the knowledge will be kept for as long as possible.' When I was young – I suppose I must have been about fourteen – every time my mother went to help someone give birth she would take me along to watch and to help. Whatever she did I put my hands over hers, and that's the way I learnt what to do."

For a pregnant woman the spirits posed something of a problem: "When an Akkha woman becomes pregnant she won't tell anyone, not even her husband. She will dress in her usual clothes and will not do anything unusual to make sure that the spirits won't notice, as if they do they might kill either the mother or the baby." Amon said that his wife didn't tell him for six months that she was pregnant, and even though he noticed he wouldn't raise the matter until she had told him. As a result, women don't go to the midwife until they are in labour and the baby is ready to come: "When the wife starts feeling the labour pains the husband will go and get the midwife if his mother or her mother aren't around. Once he's found someone to help, the husband must stay outside until the baby is born; he mustn't tell anyone what is happening so that the spirits don't know about it. When I arrive, the first thing I do is boil some water and then feel her belly so that I know when the baby will be born. When the white fluid comes out I give the mother some hot water and then say good things to her to help the baby be born very soon. The baby should be born within three days, and it's very rare that it takes longer than this. Once the baby is born I tie the cord twice with pieces of cotton and then cut in the middle with a piece of bamboo." A baby is considered to be a gift from the spirits, and it is the spirit who decides whether a woman should become pregnant or not. It seems that most women have a new baby every three years or so, although Amon did tell me of one family where a baby came along every eighteen months, which was considered most odd. If babies and children die, it is thought to be some sort of punishment from the spirits.

Midok then went on to talk about what happens if twins or a deformed baby are born. The Akkha believe that a woman should have one perfect baby and that if they have either a deformed baby or twins, the imperfections which this symbolizes will spread to the whole village, which will suffer misfortune. For this reason, twins or deformed babies are killed at birth: "Twins are a very bad fault and if they are born the midwife has to run to the headman of the village and tell him. He will take some rice husks and run to the house where the twins are and use the rice husks to stop the babies breathing. They then put the bodies in a chicken coop and if the mother is all right the father and mother take the bodies out of the village. They have to go with the headman and two magic men, as if they don't the spirits might kill them. They go into the jungle, where they have to cross a stream and make a camp there. They have to sit in this camp for the whole night and no one must sleep in case the spirits get them. In the morning the couple walk further on with the bodies; they make a trap, put the bodies in and cover them with banana leaves. Only then can they go back to the village. The next morning they go back to the trap and if they see nothing they can come back to the village to sleep. The headman and the magic men then have to do a ceremony with the couple, but they have to put a screen between them otherwise the twins become like Satan, like devils, and they could come back and kill everyone in the village.

"After this the headman and the couple go back to the stream for two more days. On the third day the villagers have to take all the couple's possessions and then burn down their house; so the couple lose everything. Then at least twenty-eight chickens have to be sacrificed as well as pigs and goats, and if the couple don't have enough animals for this, the neighbours help out by providing some more. The villagers then have to build a new house for the couple as far away from the centre of the village as possible. When the couple come back to the village they mustn't cut their hair or have a shower for a year, and they mustn't change their clothes. For a year they have to live their life apart from the rest of the village; they have to make their own path down to the water and the rice fields and married people aren't allowed to talk to them, although children and old people may do so. After all these ceremonies no one in the village can go anywhere or have any contact with anyone else for a month. If we see strangers or anyone from other villages, we just won't talk to them."

Not surprisingly, Akkha women are very scared indeed of having either twins or a deformed baby, and this was one of Ammer's constant preoccupations while she was pregnant. As she also had the knowledge that if the baby had been a girl her husband would have taken another wife, pregnancy must have been a time of considerable stress for her. There was a firm consensus in the village about the rightness of these ideas; Amon had strong feelings about wanting a son, but would not have hesitated to kill twin boys: "We love children very much indeed, but not twins or malformed babies. If we had had twin boys we wouldn't just kill one and let one live, as this would mean that terrible things could happen to the village. I would have to think about the village and what could happen if we didn't kill the babies and do the proper ceremonies." Amon said that he was willing to talk about these things only now that his son was safely born – before that there would have been a danger of the spirits killing the baby, and maybe Amon as well: "We are very scared to talk about these things; you are the first *farang* [foreigner] to whom we have told these things. They are very private to the Akkha tribe."

As we sat and talked in the dark, with the flickering oil lamps and opium pipes, the fear was palpable. The new reality with which I had just been confronted seemed only too real in the charged atmosphere, which was intensified by the darkness. This was obviously a very emotional subject, and I felt privileged that they could have trusted me enough to tell me all about it, but also a little worried lest the spirits might have been disturbed. For the rest of my time in the village I felt that I could not talk about it openly, and it was only when I had left Thailand that I was able to tell Peter what had happened.

I notice in what I have read about the Akkha that they are either roundly condemned for these "primitive and barbaric" beliefs, or this aspect of their life is not mentioned. Yet these issues are as emotionally charged in the Western world: look at any debate on abortion, amniocentesis, embryo research or how we should react to badly deformed babies. It seems to me that the difference in modern society is that we have no consensus about the view to be taken and therefore have to provide a situation in which everyone can make up their own mind about such issues according to their own conscience. In traditional Akkha society, however, there is a consensus about the rightness of their beliefs and actions, and consequently everyone is happy to abide by their traditional customs.

Next day, very regretfully, we walked under the spirit gate down the steep path away from Banghuang. I felt I had been extremely lucky here and was tremendously touched at the way the villagers had taken me into their confidence. I wondered how I was going to do justice to the reality within which Akkha women give birth, which seems so far removed from anything in the Western world.

5

TRADITION UNCHANGED:
BIRTH AMONGST THE KAREN

WE WERE ABLE TO drive the whole way to the Karen
village of Pa Pong Tam, which means literally "low village".
The track off the main road, however, was very bumpy
and we had to cross several rickety bridges and negotiate
several patches of mud before we arrived. Unlike the other
hill tribes, the Karen have lived in Thailand for a long time,
some say since the thirteenth century. They are the largest
tribal minority in Thailand and are very familiar with the
Thais, calling them *jaa*, or "old friends". Also unlike the
other groups, the Karen have a form of swidden agriculture
with rotation of crops, which means that they do not have
to move their villages very often. They tend to live at lower
altitudes than other groups with their villages, like this one,
being built on a slope close to a river at the bottom of a
valley. After the journey it seemed that we were a long way
from so-called civilization and I was therefore very surprised
when, on getting out of the van, the first thing I saw was a
children's playground. Not only was this covered with grass
and enclosed so that the animals couldn't get to it, but the
slide, swings and roundabout were all in working order.
There was also a substantial school building together with
the teacher's house and a community meeting hall. This was
clearly a village of some substance.

As we jumped out of the van we were immediately surrounded by a crowd of curious and boisterous children. After
having a good look at us – Emma's blonde hair again, coming
in for much comment – they proceeded to examine, with
great interest, everything we unpacked. Many of them were
wearing the traditional calico dress common to children of
both sexes. It is like a loose gown, made of thick unbleached
cotton, which is woven on hand looms in the village. It
starts off a bright white edged with red decorations, but
after repeated wearings and washings goes a uniform grey.
It looks as if it is almost indestructible and must be very
suitable for the village environment.

Slowly we carried all our luggage into the headman's house,
where we were going to stay. This was by far the largest
house in the village, and was made out of wooden planks
rather than bamboo like all the others. It was, however, built
in the traditional style: on stilts about ten feet off the ground.
We put all our things in what was the largest and probably
"best" room of the house, although there was nothing in it
apart from some sacks of rice being stored there. Next to
this room was a smaller one where all the family slept, and
beyond this was an open terrace, at one end of which was
the tap. For some reason, the floor around the tap was made
of split bamboo instead of wood, and as the tap tended to drip
continuously it was very wet and slippery. If I needed to use
the tap I did so very carefully, as it looked a long way to fall
to the ground below. Beyond this terrace was another small
room which, with its continually burning fire, served as the
kitchen. Unlike traditional Karen houses, this house did not
have the long windowless sloping roof; in fact it had several
windows, all of which had well-fitting shutters.

This house, the school and the playground, as well as various other improvements in the village, were a direct result of
the energy and enterprise of the headman, Bala. Amongst the
Karen being the headman is a hereditary responsibility,
although he has to have the agreement of all the other older
men in the village, not only for his election but also for his
subsequent actions. Village affairs have to be sorted out by

consensus, and headmen who are too authoritarian or otherwise unsuitable are replaced. Unless the hereditary headman can speak Thai, however, the Thai government will not recognize him as such and will appoint someone else. This person won't of course, necessarily be accepted by everyone else in the village, and it can be a source of friction, as unless the government appointee has the support of the villagers he can find it impossible to implement government policy.

In this village, however, Bala was both the hereditary headman and the government appointee, and seemed to have used his post very creatively. He had brought considerable benefits to the village, but in a way which did not disrupt traditional rhythms.

It was at his instigation that the school was built in the village, together with the house for the schoolteacher, which was used by children from all the surrounding villages. He had also managed to acquire grants for putting in a water system, and many houses had pour flush toilets after he had put one in for himself and extolled its virtues to everyone else. Thai radio has programmes in the Karen language, and as several people in the village had radios they obtained information about the outside world from this source. Bala was very keen to support many of the health suggestions made in these programmes, such as boiling drinking water and making sure that the children ate only properly cooked food. Despite these outside ideas and influences, however, the villagers seemed to be continuing with their traditional and self-contained way of life.

We had arrived mid-afternoon, so there was time to walk through the village before daylight finished. We walked up the slope straight into the middle of a herd of cows being brought in from the fields. As always, Emma enjoyed looking at the large numbers of livestock, ranging from young puppies to pigs and chickens, that wandered around at will underneath the houses. Like most Karen villages this one was on a gentle slope at the bottom of which was the river from which they would originally have obtained all their water. Only fifty or sixty years ago, Karen villages comprised one long house which was divided into several rooms and inhabited by thirty or forty people, although these have now completely disappeared and separate households are the norm.

This village had about twenty-five houses, built seemingly at random on the slope, although in actual fact they had all been carefully placed according to how they could best benefit the families who lived in them. Houses belong to the female line of the family, and the house spirit is the spirit of one of the female ancestors. The house must be placed in such a way as to benefit this spirit, and therefore the family, to the greatest degree. If the house is incorrectly placed, illness or unhappiness can result, and if a family thinks that this might be the case, they will move the house. Usually this move is only a few feet either way, but this is sufficient to change the spiritual relationships which are causing the problems. Apparently most houses in a Karen village have been moved at one time or another. Members of the same matrilineage should build their houses together, but close cousins and sisters should not have adjacent houses. Similarly, three houses should not be built in a triangular pattern equidistant from each other.

Many of the houses we passed had a small garden which was firmly fenced off from encroaching animals. Many also had granaries, and both of these had to be correctly placed to ensure that misfortune did not befall. Even the school had a garden, which looked very impressive. Dang said it was part of a government scheme to encourage villagers to grow vegetables as a cash crop rather than opium, but in fact the Karen rarely grow opium and for this reason have less cash at their disposal than most of the other groups. Their staple crop is rice, but unless they are in the lowland valleys this is hill rice, which is not grown underwater. They grow many other vegetables and also, because of the stability of their villages, various fruit trees. Although they may occasionally have a few vegetables in excess of their needs, which they may sell, they do not have a cash crop. They also raise chickens, and pigs and cows are thought to be a good and profitable investment. The Karen are known to be good elephant handlers, but as these animals have become more expensive to keep and there is less logging work for them, only a very few Karen now do this. Those who do usually provide elephant treks for tourists. Each family is totally responsible for growing their own food and making their own clothes, and we saw many women sitting on the verandas of their houses weaving the brightly coloured cloth into traditional patterns for their sarongs. While many of the adults were wearing parts of the traditional dress – maybe a sarong or a man's sleeveless top – many were also wearing the ordinary cotton sarongs and tops which constitute normal Thai dress.

After our evening meal – which for the meat eaters included the delicacy of raw pig meat mixed with herbs – we entertained a large group of children and adults by getting ready for bed. It was quite a pantomime as in the flickering light of the oil lamps we laid out our quilts, Emma taking the opportunity to play to the gallery and seemingly to keep everyone amused. I don't normally mind this at all, and I suppose I feel it's only fair that they should come along and look at me, given that I'd spent a considerable part of the day looking at them. In fact I feel quite glad that I can give them some form of entertainment! So we got ready for bed, and when it seemed there was nothing more to look at, everyone else went as well. Dang and Pascale had chosen to sleep in the kitchen area which, with the warmth from the fire, was probably the most comfortable place during this, the coldest part of the year.

We were woken just before daylight by the sound of rice being pounded, the whole house reverberating to the beat of the rice pounder, which was kept under the house. After most of the villagers had departed for their day's work in the field, leaving some of the women to get on with the domestic chores, we walked up through the village to the midwife's house. Surprisingly, she lived in one of the poorer-looking houses at the top of the village; it was made completely of bamboo instead of wood, and the roof looked in need of repair.

When I mentioned this to Dang, he said it was because she was widowed and only had two daughters, and this would mean that they had difficulty with the rice-growing and house-building. Men tend to do the heavy work in the fields and building houses, while the women concentrate on the more domestic tasks of childcare, weaving and tending to the animals and gardens. There is a considerable amount of overlap, but even so, a one-sex household such as this is at quite a disadvantage.

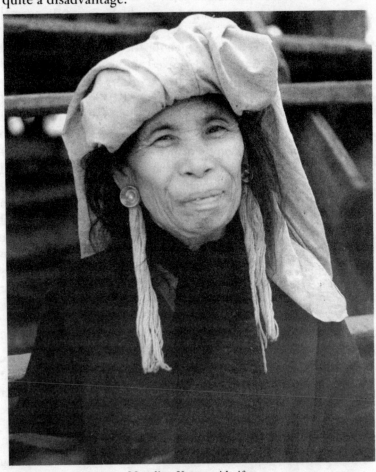

Norpli, a Karen midwife

Tradition Unchanged: Birth amongst the Karen

Norpli was a very small, wizened lady who said she was about sixty, although to me she had that look of agelessness which meant she could have been anything from forty-five to eighty. She was a widow and, like most Karen widows, lived with one of her daughters. In Karen villages there are often more widowers than widows as the women often die in childbirth, unlike villages of some other tribes where more men die younger as a result of opium addiction. Amongst the Karen, marriage is stable and divorce very uncommon. Premarital or extramarital sex is frowned upon as it is thought to bring misfortune to the village, and people who indulge may be fined, asked to marry quickly or, if none of this has any effect, made to leave the village. Dang and Bala came with me, and between them conducted the interview. At first I was very frustrated, as Norpli seemed somewhat intimidated by them and they seemed to talk more between themselves than with her. But as we continued she seemed to gain confidence and to say more, although it was very clear that most of the information about pregnancy and birth is shared by both men and women in the village, who will all have witnessed births at some time in their lives.

Norpli had been interested in the work for a long time: "When I was a little girl I used to live close to my future mother-in-law's family. She was the village midwife, and whenever she went to help someone I'd go and have a look. She taught me properly when I had my first son." It was future unhappy events, however, whch persuaded her to take on the work when she grew older: "I wanted to have lots of children, but unfortunately I wasn't very healthy. I had six, but only two are still alive. My first and second child became blind and died when they were two or three; my third I lost at six months, and my fourth was born dead. My fifth and sixth are both all right. After these experiences I decided I wanted to be a midwife to help others have healthy children. I suppose I started doing it on my own when I was about forty, and now I help with delivering about three babies a year. Mostly I help people in this village, but sometimes I'll go to other villages if their midwife is busy."

71

Norpli was summoned according to the needs of the mother: "Sometimes women may call me when they are about five months pregnant; but most of them are all right while they are pregnant and won't call me until they're ready to have the baby. Every woman knows how to look after herself when she's pregnant; if you have a daughter it's something you teach her as she grows up." This covered both the physical but also – much more importantly to the Karen – the spiritual taboos of pregnancy. They believe that pregnant women are susceptible to evil spirits entering the uterus and making them ill, so many of the taboos were to avoid this. Pregnant women should not go to a funeral in case the baby's soul is snatched to go to the afterworld with the dead person. If someone fells a tree or puts something in the path of a pregnant woman they must give the woman a chicken in recompense, otherwise the birth might be obstructed. Norpli knew of only one food taboo during pregnancy, and that was not to eat castrated pig, as this might make the baby deformed. Some Karen will not take jackfruit, as it is believed to cause contractions, as will spicy food like ginger, but not chillies. The most common reason for needing Norpli's help during pregnancy was for pain, which she would treat with massage. She said that pain at the bottom of the spine and along the top of the pelvis was very common in the last few weeks of pregnancy, but massage could easily cure this.

Birth always took place in the house, and no Karen from this village had ever given birth in hospital. Once she was called to help a woman in labour, Norpli would stay until the baby was born: "When I go to help a woman in labour, I first of all touch her belly and then I can tell whether this is the right time or not and when she is going to have the baby. Then I give her some special water to drink, over which I have said some magic words, and then I massage her and try to console her. While the mother is waiting I get her to sit upright against a sack of rice, and then I massage her. Some will be like this for three days, but usually it is only one or two days. As soon as the white fluid comes out, I know that the baby will soon be born. Then I help her to kneel up and hold on to a rope that I tie on to one of the rafters, because this is the best position in which to give birth. Then, as she pushes, I massage her stomach from behind and hold her stomach up as the baby comes out." During this period the woman would be surrounded by her family and relatives although, as Norpli put it, "Anyone can come along and have a look." Many people would give birth with the help of their mother or mother-in-law and would call Norpli only if there were problems which were difficult to deal with.

Once the baby is born the umbilical cord is quickly cut as this, according to Norpli, encourages the baby to breathe and cry: "First I tie the cord with two pieces of cotton and then I cut it with a piece of bamboo so that it is about a finger's length long. If the baby doesn't cry, I may bang on the floor to frighten it into doing so." Generally after an hour or so mother and baby are taken to the fire and the mother breastfeeds the baby. Before she does this she chews some rice and salt and puts it in the baby's mouth. This tells the baby: "I am going to feed you this milk for a year, and after that this is what you will eat." At the fire Norpli massages the mother with a hot stone wrapped in a towel, or she may make a hot compress with a towel and hot water instead: "We do this to heat and expel all the bad blood."

The husband is then responsible for dealing with the placenta. Bala demonstrated this with great delight, having had to do it four times himself for his own children: "We put the placenta and the cord in a bamboo water pipe so that the baby's heart will be cool like water and he won't get the fever. We put some banana leaves on top and then we either tie it very close to the top of a tree or bury it deep beneath the tree so that the dogs can't get at it. This is very important, as if the baby gets ill in the future this will be because one of his souls has gone away. We can ask one of the spirits to contact the cord pipe and ask the baby's soul to come back so that he will be cured."

The Karen believe that everyone has thirty-three souls which dwell in various parts of the body, the six most important being in the eyes, nose, tongue and ears. There are important souls in each wrist, and if anyone thinks that these may wander, the wrists are bound with pieces of cloth to stop this happening. If any of the souls leaves the body, illness can result, the most serious being when the souls from the ears go, which can lead to death. Souls can leave for a variety of reasons, such as being stolen by or wanting to visit a dead relative. The souls come into the body when the baby is born, and the evidence for this is in the healing of the umbilical cord. One of the souls is believed to reside in the placenta, so if it is lost – perhaps the tree is cut down, or it is taken by an animal – then a soul is lost. If a baby is ill, the parents may go to the tree where the cord is and invite the errant soul back to the baby's body. They may "buy back the soul" by offering the spirit a chicken in exchange for it.

After three days the midwife's job is considered finished and the family will kill a chicken which the midwife will then share with them: "At that time I put a white thread round the baby's wrist to keep the bad spirits away." She then receives a "payment", although it was clear that Norpli didn't view this in quite the same way as a professional midwife might do: "I'm not given any money but most people give me a new shirt, a necklace, a piece of turmeric and the leaves of seven different sorts of trees. This is just to show respect for the midwife." Norpli didn't mention a cleansing ceremony, but apparently some midwives then ritually cleanse themselves by washing their hair in water over which magic words have been said.

To the Karen the spiritual is inextricably mixed with the physical, and as Norpli discussed the way in which she dealt with any problems during pregnancy or birth, this was very evident. Although there might be practical measures to deal with problems, the spiritual aspects were equally important. Swa is the divine power who created the world together with the first man and woman, but this spirit is not interested in the affairs of men and when the Karen want help they turn to other spirits. There is a very powerful spirit called Bgha who protects all the members of a matrilineage. This may be an ancestor, commonly referred to as "the house spirit", and can be contacted for help whenever a member of the family is ill or suffering other misfortunes. Some families have a special ceremony for this spirit once a year to ward off misfortune. There is also a powerful spirit of the area who presides over the land and therefore affects the harvest, and whose help must be enlisted twice a year to ensure a good harvest. There are also various other lesser spirits of nature who are not necessarily malevolent but who could, in certain circumstances, cause harm and might have to be appeased.

Illness is thought to be a signal from the spirits that all is not well: that the spirits of the ancestors or the places are displeased or want to be fed. It is thought to be exactly the same for everyone, and although one can ignore the spirits to cure an illness, it will require more medicine than if one approached them in the first place. This is how the Karen explain why Western doctors use so many drugs! In the case of illness, the first thing to do will be to use some form of divination to determine which spirit is displeased or in some way needs to be appeased. If a person is very ill, however, normally the house spirit is the first one to be contacted. Other causes of illness might include human misdeeds such as extramarital sex, marriage with a forbidden person, wrong position of a house, and so on. It is also possible that illness could be caused by sorcery. Accident and illness are often thought to be foretold by aberrant animal behaviour, and any animals displaying such behaviour will be killed to ensure that no accident or illness befalls. There are some things, however, that cannot be changed, the most important of these being the nature and time of death. Before each person is born, he or she is asked how long they want to live and how they want to die. The Karen therefore feel that they choose the life they want and that having made their choice, they cannot then go against their destiny. However and whenever they die, it can never be untimely, as that is their choice.

Like most of the Karen, Norpli had a variety of herbal and magical cures for different problems during pregnancy. Morning sickness is not considered a problem – "It's how you know you're pregnant!" – and there is no treatment. Any problems during pregnancy, such as the constipation

I mentioned or the baby not growing well, is considered to be caused by a bad spirit. To begin with, the less powerful nature spirits are contacted: "To help cure any problem with pregnancy the family will kill a pig or a chicken (depending on the seriousness of the illness), cook it and put the meat with some rice in a bamboo pipe. We put this pipe in the jungle where the bad spirit lives, and we apologize if we have offended it in any way." If this doesn't work, the more powerful house spirit is asked for help: "We kill an even bigger chicken or pig and apologize to the house spirit. This *always* works." Similarly, Norpli used various magical cures for such things as high blood pressure: "I use a special branch which has a hole through the middle of it. I blow through the hole on to the woman's head and say some magic words, and this usually helps."

There were a variety of physical cures which Norpli used in conjunction with these spiritual/magical ones. If the baby was the wrong way round or lying awkwardly she would massage it round to the right position; in all her experience she had only ever seen three breech babies. She also had a variety of herbal cures, one of the most important being that for stopping bleeding after birth: "To stop bleeding I use the herbs blakho or puloi, which is a yellow root like turmeric. This is boiled and the water is given to the woman to drink, and that will stop it. If there is a lot of bleeding she will have to make sure that she stays near the fire and takes the herbs for two days or more, after which the bleeding will stop." At the same time the spirits would also be asked for help: "If the bleeding is very bad we will go the spirits and ask, 'Please help this woman', or maybe we will say, 'If you stop the bleeding now we will give you a pig, but if it takes as long as two days you will only get a chicken.'"

Whatever happens, however, the responsibility is not ultimately Norpli's. As Bala put it, "If the mother dies after giving birth there's nothing you can do and no one can help because it's a punishment from the spirits. We don't have any ceremonies for them or anything like that; somebody must have done something wrong, otherwise the woman wouldn't have died." Despite this somewhat fatalistic view, Bala was only too well aware of measures which had improved the health and well-being of the village; indeed he had been instrumental in seeing that they came to his village: "In the past many babies were killed by disease because it was so dirty. There was malaria and diarrhoea, but now it's cleaner and we don't suffer from these things so much. Most babies had roundworms and once they started coming out of the nose and mouth the baby would suffocate and die. This happened because we used to eat a lot of raw meat, but we are much more careful now and we don't let our children have it. We wash fruit they eat and make sure they have clean water to drink, and now everyone is much more healthy than in the past." He felt that his family exemplified this, given that all his four babies had grown into healthy children.

In a study during the early 1970s in the Karen village of Don Luang, the researchers found that the mortality rate was high, especially in infancy, and that most families lost at least one child. They also found that women were very scared of childbirth. This was true of Timet, Bala's wife, when she had her first baby: "My first birth was very painful indeed. My husband went to get the midwife, but while I was waiting the baby just came! It was very easy in the end, but at the same time I was very scared and said I wouldn't have any more." Norpli, however, felt that as most of the women worked hard, most of them had easy births: "Karen women work very hard; we have to, otherwise we have nothing to eat. I think that gives us a very hardy body so that we tend to give birth quite easily."

The Karen have no indigenous methods of contraception, so that, however frightened a Karen woman might be of giving birth, she has no option but to go on having children unless a couple decide to stop sexual intercourse. As Bala put it, "Our parents didn't know anything and would just go on having children and they'd have maybe ten or more. Maybe then they'd just stop having sex or they'd be too old to have any more." The headman himself, however, then talked about his vasectomy, which he had found out about by accident but which he obviously thought was a very good thing indeed, especially for him: "After we'd had four babies I thought that was enough. The one day when I was in the government office in town someone told me that I could have an operation so that I didn't have any more children. It seemed such a good idea that I went and had it. The official said that if I brought five more people from the village for the operation they would give me a pig, and if I found ten I would get a stereo." With his usual energy Bala recruited nine other men; probably his own enthusiasm was an important factor: "There were quite a lot of men here who didn't want any more children. When they'd had the operation they were given a T-shirt. I got a lot of ideas for the village from the government officials, and that's how we come to have the water supply and sanitation."

In contrast to Norpli, Lotyet was a vital woman of forty five who was the midwife for the village just down the road – the so-called "high village" of Pa Pong Soon. This village seemed to be perched on a very steep slope and I had great difficulty in getting down to Lotyet's house without sliding on my bottom. This was the dry season – goodness knows what happened during the rains, when presumably the slope became like a waterfall. Lotyet's house was built in the traditional pattern from bamboo, and when news of our arrival had spread throughout the village the house soon filled up with men and women who were interested to hear and see what was going on. Lotyet and her husband were very talkative, and Lotyet really seemed to enjoy telling me about her work.

She admitted to being somewhat young for this work, but had been doing it for some time: "I was about twenty-five when I started doing it on my own, but this was because the woman who taught me had died. There was no one else to do it, so I took over." There was no family connection with the work: "When I was about twenty-one or twenty-two I was pregnant for the first time and the midwife of the village came to help me. I was very interested in what she did and I asked her to teach me. I learnt a lot from my own pregnancy and I used to touch my stomach and feel the baby grow, and after I'd had the baby she went on teaching me for another two or three years. Most of the mothers who come to me come from the village, and I suppose I help about two or three mothers each year."

As she explained, not everyone in the village needed her help: "Most women in the village know how to take care of themselves when they're pregnant, and they'll come and see me only if something's wrong. Perhaps they work too hard or they have an accident, and then they'll have pain. Their husband will come and fetch me and I'll go round and see what I can do." Usually, however, women didn't contact her until they were ready to give birth. Like Norpli, she went to the woman's house and stayed with her until the baby arrived: "Wherever I go I take all my own equipment – oh yes! I'm very professional, you know."

She then showed me the rope and the piece of cloth that she proceeded to tie up to one of the low beams in the house. Everyone then looked with great interest as I had a go at hanging on the rope and feeling what it would be like to give birth in this position. I was very surprised at how comfortable it was. I had thought that the rope would be most unsteady and that I would wobble around and feel quite unsupported, but the opposite was the case. I could get myself into a variety of different positions, and somehow hanging on to the rope was quite relaxing and yet stable at the same time. Lotyet then got behind me and showed me how she would hold a woman as she pushed the baby out. This was yet another source of steadiness, although I would think that for some people the presence of another person quite so close could be offputting. Nevertheless it would feel like a joint effort, and I think I would have felt very supported in every way.

Once the baby was born, Lotyet followed the same processes as Norpli in cutting the cord and then putting the placenta in a bamboo pipe. Lotyet's husband explained what he did when he took the placenta out to a tree: "When the husband goes out to put the pipe in a tree he will also cut a stick from a tree or a bush. If the baby is a girl he will give the

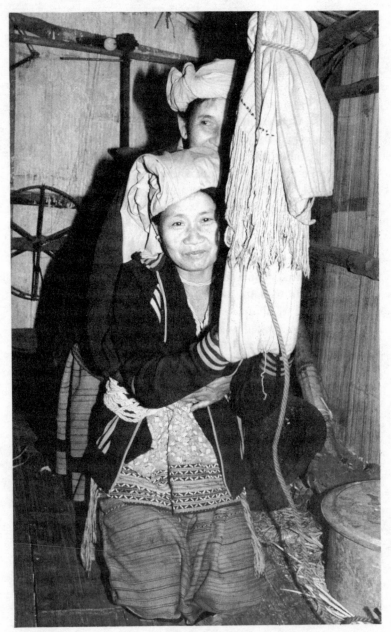

Giving birth, Karen style

stick to her as a weaving stick [the stick used in a loom to pull the weft firmly] so that when she grows up she will become an expert weaver. If the baby is a boy the stick will be given to him as a gun so that he will grow up to be a good hunter. Then the stick will be left in the house somewhere as the baby grows up."

Families were having fewer children now: "In the past, if a family didn't have ten or more children it was not a happy family, as it needed that number of people to tend the rice fields, cut the wood and do all the necessary jobs. Right now about four or five is the best number" – although no one could explain why this was so. It was still important to have a mix of sexes, however: "The best thing is to have an equal number of boys and girls. If you have all girls you have lovely clothes but everyone is thin because there is no food. If you have all boys you live in a big house and have lots of rice but everything is dirty and no one has any decent clothes to wear."

After the birth of the baby the mothers in this village ate only rice and salty water for a month. Lotyet would not visit the mother again after birth unless she had any problems. For women who had difficulty with breastfeeding, the father would go out and get a banana blossom which he would cook and give to his wife. Apparently this always worked very well. There was no exclusion period but Lotyet said that most women would stay around the house for a month, although this depended on how they felt and the needs of the family: "Usually after giving birth the women don't do any hard work or go to the fields for a month, but it depends on how healthy they are. There are some women who get up quickly and go to the rice fields and they're perfectly happy, while others need to rest for longer." Unlike the headman of the previous village, Lotyet's husband felt that people weren't as healthy as they used to be: "In the old days when women became pregnant there was not much sickness. When a woman had a child she stopped for just a couple of days before going back to work again. I think that people were much more healthy then."

This could, of course, have been a sentimental harking back to the "good old days", but he had interesting reasons for saying this: "The birds and pigs that we eat aren't so healthy now. They eat chemicals and the air and water isn't so good as it used to be. Nowadays there seems to be a lot of disease, a lot more than there used to be."

The Karen have a strong feeling that they are a part of nature, as exemplified in one of their sayings: "We are the same as a tree. We are born, we grow old as a tree or an animal does. Men are the same thing. Me, you, the Thai and others; we are all made the same way." With this in mind they have a very non-exploitative way of dealing with the environment, and they have all sorts of sayings describing how the earth should be used. These range from general ideas about how the crops should be sown and how humans should deal with animals, to more specific items such as how many trees should be felled to make a field. I tried to find out how Lotyet's husband got to know about the chemicals and whether this related to the local activities of a company or government department, but without success. As we drove back to the village, however, it was clear that there was very little forest left, and perhaps watching this destruction had shown him that his age-old balance with the environment was being destroyed.

PART II

TRAVELLING IN INDONESIA

6

ขๅ ๓

INTO INDONESIA

BEFORE I CAME to this part of the world I had never appreciated the size and scale of Indonesia, consisting as it does of 13,000 islands which stretch for 5,000 kilometres from the Asian mainland to the Pacific Ocean. This enormous country has a population of 156 million which is expected, despite the best efforts of the government birth control programme, to increase to 200 million by the end of the century. There are numerous languages and ethnic groups as well as a phenomenal array of natural resources which, since the sixteenth century, have been a magnet for European entrepreneurs. Indonesia was ruled by the Dutch for 350 years and gained independence in 1945. Since then, despite various political upheavals, the country has managed to keep its diverse groups intact within a national identity.

In the eight weeks that a visitor is allowed to stay in Indonesia it is obviously impossible to do any more than just scratch the surface. This was especially true for us, as we didn't have the money to fly, which is the only way of travelling the vast distances in this country in a reasonable amount of time. Travelling by boat and overland, we visited three different places which were neither particularly "out of the way" nor off the tourist tracks (this would have taken too much time to achieve) but which, fortuitously, showed me three very different practices of traditional birth and mid-wifery. We took with us Letchimi, the Malaysian friend who had helped with my interviewing in Malaysia and did the same in Indonesia, where the language is very similar. This was as much an adventure for her as it was for us, as she had never been out of Malaysia before.

We began by going to Sumatra, the second largest island in Indonesia. It is sparsely populated – large areas are still covered with jungle – and is only now starting to be exploited for its natural resources. Going the cheapest way – by boat from Penang in Malaysia – we ended up in Medan, a noisy, stinking place which I hated and thought was the supreme example of what you get when self-interested capitalism is allowed to run rife with no regard for the social consequences of individual action. There is a great feeling of busyness and moneymaking, borne out by the streets of shops, hotels and various new buildings springing up everywhere. The place seems, however, to have an unfinished air about it, with roads that peter out towards the edges into puddles and potholes instead of pavements. Every morning oil drums are set up in the middle of the road in an attempt to keep the traffic in disciplined lanes, but by the end of the day most of these have been knocked over and the traffic continues on its haphazard way, pouring out fumes and smoke which hang like fog in the air, making it feel even more suffocatingly hot. The way the motorcycle rickshaw drivers drive seems to me symptomatic of the whole Medan ethos. These vehicles, which sound like an angry lawn mower, think nothing of driving on the wrong side of the road against all the oncoming traffic if they think it will make it easier for themselves, or to make a little extra money.

With the heat, fumes and noise of Medan, whatever sanguinity I might have possessed evaporated rapidly and we decided to go to Lake Toba as soon as possible. At the bus station we were badly hustled by a couple of lads who dragged our things away from us and demanded the extortionate sum of Rp50,000 for a bus journey that should have cost only Rp8,000. Once we had rumbled what they were up to, the lads refunded the excess money without any embarrassment. I suppose they thought we were rich foreigners and a soft touch, and perhaps they get away with it often enough to make it worthwhile – the only reason we realized was that it seemed rather expensive, so we checked in the guidebook what the price should be. That sort of thing always leaves a nasty taste in my mouth, as I hate going around not trusting people, assuming that I am going to be ripped off, and therefore bargaining hard over every rupiah. It's hardly the way to enjoy travelling around a country. I also find it hard to accept that there are people around who will take advantage of my naivety or lack of information in this very calculating way.

By rushing on to the bus as soon as it arrived in the station we managed to get a proper seat, although by the time the bus was full, with people sitting on extra seats at the back and front and standing jam-packed in the gangway, I couldn't see much except out of the side window. In the event this was probably just as well as the driver drove like a madman, hooting at everything in sight, although whether this was just a friendly greeting or to make everyone move out of his way I preferred not to know or see. The road to Lake Toba is better than many in Sumatra which, in spite of recent improvements, is still a difficult place to get around. Roads and bridges tend to get washed away in the wet season and are then patched up for the dry season, when they are bumpy and uncomfortable. There always seem to be more people wanting to travel than there is transport to take them, and in consequence buses are always crammed full. Time and again, however, I realized that in Sumatra there is no such thing as a full bus. However uncomfortably one is sitting (or standing or squatting or clinging on to something) and however much one can't envisage how another person can possibly get in, there is *always* room for one more person and their boxes, bags and livestock.

Halfway there a lot of the passengers disembarked and we breathed more freely for a few minutes until they were replaced by even more people. Someone tried to push themselves on to our seat, which would have meant that I would have had to have Emma on my lap. After our experience at the bus station and paying full fare for Emma, I wasn't going to have it and just sat tight until he went off somewhere else! The bus resumed its journey, plunging along the road which winds up on to a plateau of undulating hills and then down to Lake Toba, providing a fabulous view of the lake. The hills around the lake and on Samosir, the island in the lake, are almost bare except for a few pine trees, giving it a very open feeling compared with the profusion of trees and plants in the lowlands from which we had come.

Getting out of the bus, we were immediately assailed by the freshness of the air at this higher elevation. This place is well frequented by Western travellers and I was therefore quite surprised when we were surrounded by an interested group of people who just seemed to want to stand and look at us. Once they realized that Letchimi was Malaysian, she was besieged with questions. What was Malaysia like? How easy or difficult would it be to get a job there? How much money could they expect to earn? For many Indonesians Malaysia is an eldorado, a reasonably accessible place to which they can go to earn unimaginable amounts of money. They are interested in Western countries, but they must seem as inaccessible as the moon, as few ordinary Indonesians could ever hope to save up the money to go there, much less live there.

We allowed ourselves to be ushered into the next boat going across the lake to the island of Samosir and were treated to some beautiful close-harmony singing by a group of young people who seemed to be doing it just for their own pleasure. It sounded very Latin American but could equally well have been local Batak folk songs or Indonesian pop music. At this time of year the winds can make the lake quite choppy, and with the music seeming to match the motion of the boat it was a very pleasant ride. Unfortunately we didn't end up where we had hoped and had to disembark at Tuk

Tuk, the main centre for Western visitors on the island. As I went to bed that night and listened to the sounds of Western pop music and revelry wafting up from the little restaurant below, traditional midwives seemed a long, long way away.

7

WHEN THE SPIRIT MOVES: MIDWIFERY AND SHAMANISM AMONGST THE BATAKS

As I HAD suspected, since Tuk Tuk had been built as a stopping place for Westerners there were no traditional midwives living nearby. Asking around about this, however, I did have a very interesting discussion with Mark, the son of our *losman* (guesthouse) owner. He was married to a teacher on the mainland, where she worked during the week while he stayed with his father, helping out in the restaurant and looking after the children. He certainly seemed to be very involved with them, as nearly every time I saw him he was either carrying the youngest one around or playing with the older one.

Mark explained how he had helped his wife during both her pregnancies with a variety of traditional and Western approaches: "She went to see the doctor regularly to get these injections to make her strong. She had ten in all, and they cost me Rp50,000." This must have represented a considerable amount of money to two young people who would not have been earning very much, so I asked him why she had to have the injections and what they were: "She needed the injections to make her strong; they are special injections that the doctor gives."

Whatever could they have been? For that extortionate price I hope they were more than just iron or vitamins, which could have been given in the first place. These injections, however, seemed to come into the same "necessary" category as some of the more traditional practices to ensure that his wife would be all right: "After she had given birth I made up a fire under her bed to keep her warm and made sure that she had lots of chicken so that her milk was good." He also said that he helped with all the washing, which he described as "very dirty", although I don't know how characteristic he was of a modern Batak man in helping with this chore. He had an unquestioning attitude that whatever the doctor did must be right, just as he also believed that certain traditional practices like the fire were also necessary. By using both he felt he had ensured the best possible outcome for his wife.

Tuk Tuk had obvious limitations, so the next day we walked over to Tomok to find Mongoloi, who, according to both the guidebook and Robin Hanbury-Tenison (the explorer and founder of Survival International), was an invaluable source of information about Batak life. As we walked along tracks, footpaths and finally the main road into Tomok, I kept thinking that I could have been in Scotland. The hills, although not high, were bare and sometimes craggy, bisected with gullies which in the wetter times of the year would be filled with water. Patches of straggling pine trees added to the illusion, and only the remains of the rice terraces reminded me where we were. These hills, which run in a ridge down the whole length of the island, are the edge of the volcano which erupted in the middle of the lake and from which the island of Samosir was formed. This island is in the middle of Lake Toba, a huge lake 56 miles long and 19 miles wide, the largest in Sumatra. Samosir wasn't discovered by a Westerner until 1853, when it was connected to the mainland by a narrow isthmus of land. As it was so inconvenient not to be able to sail all the way round, the Dutch built a canal through the isthmus to give Samosir its present island status.

We had arrived during the dry season when all the water courses were dry and often stuffed full of plastic bags and bottles as well as other rubbish. The earth looked as if it was

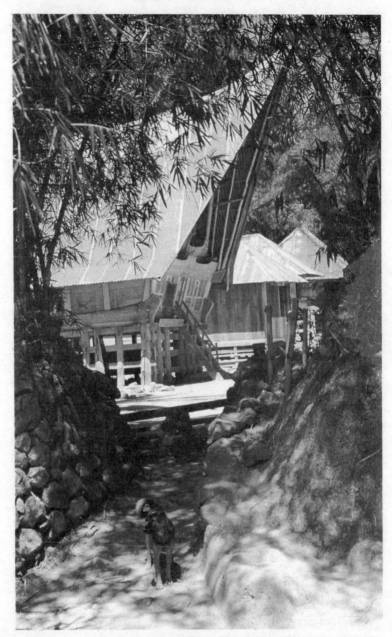

The entrance to a Batak village

as hard as iron, and I was surprised to see farmers breaking it up with their hoes. Lifting the hoe high above their heads and smashing it on to the unyielding ground in a slow-motion rhythm looked like backbreaking work. I couldn't understand why they didn't wait for the rainy season when the earth would be soft and easier to plough, but found out later that they were getting the soil ready to plant peanuts, which are an important crop grown during the dry season when the land is not required for growing rice. Where there is a spring, or where the farmer can afford a pump to pump water out of the lake, rice can be grown all year round, but few farmers do this.

In the past, Batak civilization was greatly influenced by the Hindus, who introduced wet rice culture as early as the sixteenth century. This more efficient and effective method of growing rice made them relatively prosperous and able to support a dense population. Until the late nineteenth century the Bataks were relatively isolated in their highlands, yet they had a strong culture and their own form of literacy. As a group they were feared and left alone by the lowlanders, partly because of their relative isolation and partly because of their reputation for ferocity and cannibalism. To a Batak a stranger equalled an enemy; therefore direct contact with the outside world was avoided. Even amongst themselves paths and bridges were not constructed or maintained between villages, as there was considerable fear and animosity between different groups.

The Batak men spent a lot of time at war, which broke out on any pretext and led to bloody feuds between villages. It was often the primary activity for the men, who left most of the domestic work and growing of food to the women. There were many regulations about the conduct of war, in particular that women and children could not be taken captive or eaten, which was probably just as well or the group could easily have become extinct. Captured enemies, along with traitors and those who had committed adultery with certain of the higher classes of women, were categories of individuals who could be eaten. This was a very grisly business, but the Bataks believed that it was the only way to prevent the soul of such persons from doing further damage. If a wrongdoer was eaten by everyone in the village, his soul was rendered powerless and no further harm could come to anyone there.

This cannibalism fascinated the first Europeans who visited the Bataks, as from an anthropological point of view they were unique in having a culture and being literate, yet still being cannibals. It was during the nineteenth century that their isolation ended when Islam spread to the Bataks around Lake Toba through the efforts of the German Rheinische Mission. Now about one-third of the Bataks are Christian, one-third are Muslim and one-third are pagan. Since then cannibalism has, of course, been abolished, although when Robin Hanbury-Tenison visited them in the early 1970s he heard of a case where a Batak boy had been executed and two others gaoled for the ritual killing and eating of a girl from another group.

Nowadays the Bataks are one of the largest cultural minorities in Indonesia, numbering around one and a half million people, most of whom live in a wide area around Lake Toba. They are still basically an agricultural community, and although swidden culture is used by some groups living on poorer soil, those who live around Lake Toba use wet rice culture. They also grow a wide range of vegetables as well as raising cattle, oxen and horses. Those who live by the lake also fish, and fish is an important part of the Batak diet. As with many agricultural groups there is no possession of land and it cannot be given away, sold or pawned. Possession is gained only by cultivation and this use, rather than the land itself, is inherited from the family of the first cultivator. Traditionally the Bataks also had a number of industries which included traditional metalwork, wood-carving, canoe-making and work in bone shell and bark. Some of the traditional houses still bear witness to this, but this sort of work can mostly now be found only in the tourist shops.

We found Mongoloi's house, which was far more modest than the guidebook suggested, having only two places available in which to stay. One of these was a thatched traditional house, the other was a traditional rice barn which had been built on to the house in which Mongoloi and his family lived.

We sat in a room underneath the rice barn and admired the huge pillars, on each of which a large round slab of wood prevented stop the mice from crawling up and eating the rice which would have been stored in the room above. Mongoloi didn't think there would be any problems in finding traditional midwives who, he said, were still often used, despite the existence of a hospital and several clinics around the island. His wife, Uli, had in fact used the local midwife for the birth of their fourth child five years ago. We decided then and there to stay with Mongoloi, as although many tourists come to Tomok, it is one of the main transport centres and therefore a very good base for getting around the rest of the island.

Two days later, having settled ourselves into Mongoloi's accommodation, we went to see Anton Ompung. She lived in a village about a mile down a small track which started at the side of Mongoloi's house and meandered through the fields towards the hills at the back. We walked past the dry rice fields, most of which had already been broken up in readiness for the planting of peanuts. Many people did not like this dry season as it meant that little work could be done in the fields, and no one liked the winds which came at this time of the year. These winds were certainly very eerie and kept me awake on several nights, and Uli told me that a lot of people suffered from colds and flu on account of the weather.

In several of the fields we passed stone buildings which, Mongoloi told us, were the traditional graves of the Bataks. Each family would have a grave built on the family land which consisted of a hollow square base made out of bricks or concrete in which would be put the bones of dead family members. Before the coming of Christianity a model of a Batak boat or a house would be constructed on the top, but these pagan artefacts had given way to more Christian models and designs. Members of the family who had moved away from the family land, sometimes to other far-flung parts of Indonesia, would nevertheless arrange for their bones to be brought to rest in the family grave.

The village, when we arrived, was surrounded by a mud wall on which grew a thick bush of bamboo. There was a gap in the wall in which was a "gate" consisting of several upright pieces of bamboo knocked into the ground. The animals, mainly pigs, had a horizontal piece of wood slung round their necks which stopped them from being able to walk between the uprights of the gate. Unfortunately it was at about knee level, so to avoid their legs being continually knocked by the wood they had to walk around with mincing steps, which made them look as if they were dancing about the compound. As this village was very small it had only one row of houses, only one of which was built in the traditional style with a saddleback roof. As far as I could see it did not have the traditional communal hall or rice barns. According to Mongoloi the water for this village came from a well that frequently dried up during this season. No wonder there was a continuous procession of people going past Mongoloi's house with water carriers, presumably taking the water from the lake and carrying it a mile or more to this village.

We sat in the cool gloom of Anton Ompung's house to talk and were joined by several other women suckling babies and children from breasts that looked even more diminished than mine, which had got that way after four years of feeding Emma. They all joined in giving me the benefit of their opinions and experience. Anton was in her sixties but still delivering several babies each year in this village, where everyone wanted as many children as they could to help on the land. It was Anton who told me how Batak midwives are introduced to their calling: "I didn't learn what to do as a midwife from anyone. I got the blessing from a dream. In my dream I saw an old woman with a cloth tied over her head; she gave me a chicken's egg and blessed me. She told me that she was blessing me to be a midwife, and then she gave me the egg. Since I had the dream I have known how to deliver babies. I had this dream about twenty-five years ago when I became a widow, and ever since then I have been helping women with deliveries."

It was only later that I realized the significance of this initiation and the name which these traditional midwives have, which is *"si baso huta"*. *Huta* is the Batak word for village, and I assumed that *si baso* was the Batak word for midwife, but in fact it means shaman. The original Batak shamans were always female and were capable of going into a trance when the spirit of an ancestor or some other spirit would enter them, so that the villagers could talk directly with the spirit. The dream initiation and the name are all that remain of this past. None of the midwives referred to this heritage – whether because they did not know about it or because they were ashamed of it in the light of their Christian teaching I do not know. They were converted such a short time ago that I find it hard to believe they have actually forgotten, but sometimes in the fervour of being converted, and in their desire to show that they really are converted, such knowledge is conveniently "forgotten" until much later when, being more confident about their professed beliefs, they can turn back to and use this old knowledge. I wondered also whether the fact that Mongoloi was a well-known practising Christian made Anton unwilling to talk in too much detail about it.

She continued to talk quite comfortably, however, about her "dream woman" as if she were a friend: "I still have contact with the woman who first came to me in the dream. If I need something or if I need help, the woman will come to me again in a dream. No one in my family has ever been a *bidan* before, and I don't teach my children. To be a *bidan* you have to be blessed by the spirit, as I was, in a dream. Then nothing can go wrong." I found it hard to believe that this was all that had to happen and that no further practical knowledge was obtained before practising, but other midwives confirmed this was true. In fact, like Anton, most of them said it was something that could not be taught and that in any case the help of the dream woman was necessary to ensure that they were blessed to do the work and that everything would always go well.

As in so many other traditional villages, pregnant women came to Anton only if they felt there was a problem that required her expert assistance: "When women are pregnant they call me when they need my services. It depends – sometimes when they are two months pregnant they may call me, or when they are six or seven months. Sometimes when they feel that the baby is not in the right position they will call me so that I can put it back. I use coconut oil to do the massage." Anton said that in her experience the healthier a woman was, the less she would need to do for her during pregnancy. Traditionally there used to be various pregnancy taboos, such as not sitting in the doorway of a house too long so that the birth canal keeps clear, and it was also believed that towards the end of pregnancy the husband should stay with his wife, especially at night when, if she had bad dreams, the spirits might upset the new baby. No one, however, mentioned any of these beliefs being practiced now.

Once the woman went into labour, Anton would go to her house and stay there for as long as necessary until the baby was born: "During the delivery I'll stay one night, or half a day, or sometimes only a few hours. It all depends on what the woman needs. The position in which she gives birth depends on her. Normally they lie down, but sometimes they are on their knees and sometimes they hold on to a rope." Once the baby is born and the placenta is delivered, the umbilicus is cut. Anton used to do this with a piece of bamboo but now uses a blade, putting areca nut oil on the cut to ensure that there is no infection: "We break open the areca nut and take out the white kernel inside. We then squeeze it with bamboo to make a black oil, which we use to massage the navel." In this community, areca nut is a cure-all for many things: "Areca nut is good medicine for children; they can eat it when they have a fever. If the child's head is soft you can just bite the nut and rub it on the soft part." Mongoloi also told me about several dishes which could be made using areca nut that should be eaten regularly to keep one healthy. Once the placenta is delivered it is buried, then a banana tree is planted on top of it.

Traditionally after the birth of a child the house was taboo to others for seven days, but in this village help was provided from other women: "Once the baby is born close relatives or neighbours will come to stay and watch over the woman at night. We do this for at least seven nights to help the mother and make sure that she doesn't roll over the baby. During this time the mother also sits near the fire to make sure that she keeps warm, maybe for one or two weeks depending again on how healthy she is and how much she needs it. At the same time she should also take a lot of the bangun-bangun leaf for the breastmilk, and chicken meat to get her strength back. If there is any difficulty with the breastmilk flowing, we heat up betel leaf over a hot fire and then rub it on the breast. If the baby dies we do this so that all the milk comes out." Usually after two weeks the mother would go back to the fields to work, but again this would depend on her health as well as the needs of her family. After seven days there would be a small celebration for everyone, with a shared meal of chicken. Anton told me this was called the "closing of the watch" day and signified that it was no longer necessary for anyone to stay with the mother.

Anton said that Batak women were strong and rarely had problems with birth, although she had a whole range of herbal remedies should they be necessary. It seemed, however, that these cures were all well known, and Mongoloi was able to tell me about a huge range of remedies which he said he had learnt from his mother and which most Bataks knew about. These included cures for simple problems like stomach ache as well as more exotic diseases like malaria and snake bite. These local remedies were generally tried before going to the doctor. Anton did not charge for her services: "I don't charge women a particular fee. They pay me with chickens or rice or anything according to their means." She delivered three or four babies each month, and as she said, "Here in the rural areas no one controls birth and we have as many babies as we can, as we need more children to work in the fields. Yes, you can control birth in the cities, but not here."

As we walked back, Mongoloi told us something about "the old religion" from which the dreams of these midwives originated, although it was clear that his Christianity meant that he was not quite comfortable when confronted with these beliefs. This religion was strongly related to Hindu ideas, with the world divided into three sections: an upper world of seven spheres, which was the home of the gods and their families; the middle world, which belonged to man; and the underworld of the dead, ghosts and demons. It was believed that formerly heaven was very close to earth and there was regular communication between the two. Human pride destroyed this relationship, and since then the gods have lost interest in mankind, who turn to them only at times of direst need.

The god of all was known as Mula Djadi na Bolon; he lived in the highest heaven, was not concerned about the affairs of earth, and did not receive any direct honour or sacrifice. Instead of a wife this god had a blue chicken which laid three eggs, from which hatched three gods, which lived one level lower and were worshipped as a trinity. There was also an evil divinity called Naga Padoha, a serpent who, when he eventually broke loose, would be responsible for the ultimate destruction of the world. To the Bataks, however, the most important spirits were the departed ancestors or *begu*, who had to be propitiated regularly with sacrificial ceremonies by descendants to ensure the good fortune of the family. A *begu* who had attained a revered and exalted status in the underworld by virtue of the sacrifices provided by the living could be extremely helpful in combating a host of lesser ghosts and malevolent spirits.

While any male family member could provide the necessary sacrifices and rites for satisfying the *begu*, male priests or *datu* would be used for anything more complicated. These were always male and were specialists in occult knowledge, learnt through a rigorous apprenticeship which included divination, the making of protective talismans, and sorcery. The *si baso huta* or shaman was nearly always a woman who, through being able to go into a trance, enabled people to commune directly with spirits; she was often employed in the case of illness. The Bataks also had a large number of religious artefacts, some of which belonged to the priest but some of which belonged to the village. Most of the tourist and souvenir shops are festooned with replicas of many of these religious items, which are all that remain of them nowadays.

For the average Batak, however, the most important aspect of their religion, apart from the *begu*, was the *tondi* or soul substance which was enjoyed by men, animals, rice and iron implements. This originated while the baby was still inside the mother, and its nature determined the future lot of the person. It existed near the body – if it left this caused illness, and if it left for ever, death would occur; then it would become a *begu* or ancestral spirit. Much effort was required from a person to keep the *tondi* in good humour and therefore·close to the body. Improving one's lot in this world could be done only by nourishing the *tondi* and guarding it, especially by eating one's enemies so that their *tondi* became neutralized and couldn't negatively affect anyone else's. As well as sacrificing to *begu*, sacrifices might also be made to the *tondi* of dangerous wild animals or plants (to ensure a good crop), as well as to useful inanimate objects. At times of special crisis the priest would carry out these rites on behalf of families or larger social units. Women who died in childbirth were considered to have committed some crime against their *tondi* to the extent that it no longer wished to stay by their bodies. Those who died in this dishonourable way would be thrown under the house and burnt.

Through a series of lucky coincidences I met Nailialang, who was expecting her eighth child. Although she had decided to have her baby in the hospital in Amberita (a largish place by Batak standards) she was also getting the help of the local *si baso huta*. We sat sipping coffee in her brother's restaurant while, looking exhausted, she told us about her marital problems. Earlier in the pregnancy she had wanted to separate from her husband, but for Batak women this is extremely difficult to do. Before the coming of Christianity, women were considered to be first the property of their father and later the property of their husband and, if he died, the property of another male relative. The status of the woman depended on the status of the man responsible for her. There were various rules about who could marry whom, and many

101

women would be expected to marry certain men because of the family relationship they had with each other. If a woman became pregnant without being able to marry she could be forced to marry a man of lower rank, although women did have various means of forcing guilty lovers into marriage and apparently frequently did so.

Polygamy used to be allowed and Mongoloi told me that Uli's grandfather had had three wives, although only the richer families were able to afford this. Divorce could be obtained only at the instigation of the man, with the children staying with the husband. It seemed to me that these ideas were still very strong as Nialialang explained how she had wanted a divorce from her husband, but as this was almost unheard of in the Batak community, she had been forced to stay with him. She said that the only grounds for divorce could be if the woman didn't give birth to a son: "We Batak people prefer sons to daughters because sons carry on the family name. Even just having one son is enough to carry the family name. If a woman doesn't give birth to a son, the father-in-law will advise the son to marry another woman to have a son. The first wife will still be taken care of by the husband."

Sialliagan, who was Nailialang's *si baso huta*, arrived somewhat out of breath, having come quickly from the river where she had been doing her washing. She was much younger than Anton but had been practising for eleven years or so. She still had a lot of work to do, despite the fact that many of the Amberita mothers went to the clinic for regular checkups and some actually had their babies there. Most women came to her for massage both before and after birth, and many used her services for the birth as the government midwife wasn't necessarily always available. Like Anton, she had become a midwife as the result of a dream: "I didn't learn how to be a midwife from anyone, it came naturally. Once I had a dream where an old woman came and blessed me and gave me some oil and also put some oil on me. From that day onwards I became a midwife. In those days I really enjoyed being a midwife, which is why I was blessed by the old woman."

102

After a while, however, she had become tired of the demands of the work: "I was a midwife for a long time and then I got tired of the job because people came calling at odd hours; sometimes they came at two or three o'clock in the morning. So I decided to stop doing it, but when I did I became very ill. There was something on my neck, a tumour-like thing. I went to the hospital and had an operation, but even so I was still very ill and I could hardly move for about six months." She showed us the scar on her neck and said that even as a result of an operation and various hospital treatment she had not felt well and had decided to recontact her spirit from the dream: "I called back the spirit and told her that I would continue being a midwife and promised not to give up again. Only then did I recover from my illness. So you see, I can't give up being a midwife even if I wanted to, because if I did I would be ill again." Since that time, however, she had found her work very fulfilling and was extremely happy with it. As she said, "Not everyone can be a midwife and I am blessed for doing it."

Like Anton, Sialliagan usually saw mothers during their pregnancy, those going to the hospital for checkups being as keen to see her as those who didn't: "When women are expecting a baby they will come to see me in my house or I go to see them; it all depends in which month of pregnancy they call me. Sometimes they call to see me so that I can tell them whether they are pregnant or not. I can tell by feeling even if the woman is only one month pregnant. Also if they want I can do the massage for them before giving birth. Naihailang is coming to me twice a week for massage even although she is giving birth in the hospital. It all depends on what the woman wants. If the baby is in the wrong position I will massage with special coconut oil and put it back in the right position." In spite of having the clinic nearby, most women gave birth at home unless they had particular problems, and while some would call the hospital midwife, others would call Sialliagan.

Also, she cut the umbilical cord with bamboo and buried the placenta, but felt that the position in which women now gave birth had been influenced by the doctors at the clinic: "Nowadays when giving birth we lie down, but in the olden days the

Bataks used to hold on to a rope and kneel. They lie down to give birth because the doctor from the hospital comes to the village and tells them to do so." She seemed just to accept that this was the way things had changed, and I think I would have had to talk to her for much longer and get to know her much better before she would have been willing to tell me what she really thought about it.

Sialliagan continued to be involved with mothers after the birth, wherever it had taken place: "After the birth the mother doesn't take chillies for a while, she takes bangun-bangun and lots of water. She'll also eat lots of sour things to make her thirsty, because drinking a lot at this time is very good for the mother. For one month or more, depending on the mother's health, I'll do the *mendedang*, which is keeping a slow fire going for the mother to sit beside. This keeps her body warm and is also very healthy, especially for her hips. She'll lie down beside the fire for an hour or two each day; it depends on how she feels. After the birth, for two months I'll do the massage for her to put the body back to its normal position again. Also this will help to cleanse her inside, in that when she gets her period everything will come out."

Sialliagan also had in common with Anton a variety of herbal remedies for various problems, with the areca nut much in evidence. She had not heard of the "closing of the watch" ceremony, saying the only ceremony she knew of for newborn babies was that of Christian baptism. Unlike Anton, she carried out other healing work as well as midwifery: "I massage others as well as pregnant women, like if someone falls or has a sprain they will come to me for massage. I also give medicine for stomach ache and other similar pains which is made from pounded herbs over which I say some prayers. I also work in the fields growing onions and peanuts." In a year she said she delivered about seven babies.

We caught up with Nail Helpin as she was hurrying to the house of a little girl suffering from what Uli said was flu induced by the winds. Nail Helpin was a vital woman in her mid-thirties who later told us that she had given birth to six children of her own. She massaged the child, who cried bitterly the whole time because apparently her family had been teasing her and saying that we might take her away with us! After the massage, when I took a Polaroid picture of her with her family, she had quietened down quite a lot, so I hope it wasn't too traumatic for her.

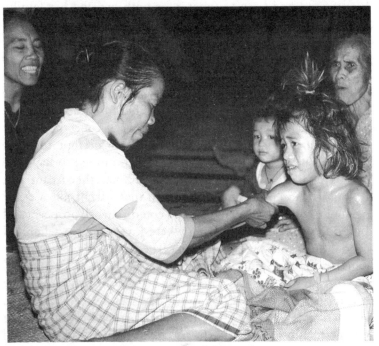

Nail Helpin massaging a child with fever

We started to talk to Nail Helpin after the massage, but as she didn't like talking in front of so many people we talked to her later at her house, which was in a beautiful setting right down by the lake. I thought at first that this was the midwife who had helped Uli, but apparently they were just good friends. As well as being a midwife Nail Helpin was also a general healer, particularly experienced in dealing with sprains and bone injuries. She told us about the different sorts of massage she used and the recipes for several herbal preparations which she put on the injury after the massage, all made out of easily obtainable things like eggs, tamarind and coconut oil and well-known herbs. For the little girl, the oil (specially formulated for a fever) had contained onion, garlic and ginger, together with fourteen other herbs.

Like all the other midwives Nail Helpin had come into the work through a dream, but this had started very early in her life and had been traumatic for both her and her family: "When I was about six years old I had a dream in which an old woman (I don't know her name, but she is supposed to be the first medicine woman and I call her my Nenek) appeared and pressed my forehead. When I woke up I had a scar on my forehead and it's still there today, as you can see." There were indeed two marks on each side of her forehead, about the size of a fingerprint. Her family were very concerned about the dream and shaved off her hair in an attempt to make sure that all evil was cast off, but she continued to have the dream regularly: "When I got older I still had this dream, but I wouldn't accept it, and it was then that I went like a crazy person. I couldn't sleep in peace, I couldn't work properly and I used to walk off not knowing where I was going or where I'd been." Her family were very concerned and gathered relatives together for a meeting. Music was played and Nail Helpin told the "dream woman" that she would accept whatever it was she had for her: "From that day onwards I was perfectly all right, and when I was about twenty I got married. After having my first baby I had the dream again and the woman told me to start practising massage, and until today this is what I have done."

It was obvious that the dream woman was a constant companion: "When a sick person comes to me for a cure, before I go to bed I'll think of her and ask Nenek how I should cope. Either that or I take a betel leaf and hold it between my hands on my forehead and explain to her that I need her help with someone. Then, when I'm in a deep sleep, Nenek will come to me and she'll tell me not only what herbs I should use but where I'll find them in the jungle. The next day I go to get the herbs where she told me to go and then I'll prepare the medicine and the person will be cured. I always get the help of the dream woman before making any medicine, as I don't know how to do it on my own." Nail Helpin was proud of her expertise and her ability as a healer and described two occasions when seemingly hopeless cases had been cured. One of these was her own child, who had a bad accident; the other was a pregnant woman who had been told by the doctors at the hospital that her baby was dead. In each case Nenek had come to her in a dream and given her specific instructions as to what she should do; as a result her child had been cured and the baby was born alive.

Nail Helpin helped women in childbirth in much the same way as the other midwives I'd spoken to, but explained in greater detail about the special food and sitting by the fire. This was done to ensure that all the blood was expelled after the birth so that the woman wouldn't have any problems with infection. She said it also meant that the woman would be much healthier when she returned to the fields to work. She also said that women did not have breastfeeding problems if they massaged their breasts and made sure that everything flowed properly, although if by any chance there were problems she used the same herbal remedies as the others. Similarly with breech deliveries; there were almost unheard of and wouldn't happen if the woman came to Nail Helpin for massage to ensure that the baby was in the right position for birth. Like Sialliagan she found that women now gave birth "the modern way" on their backs, rather than kneeling and holding on to a rope.

Unlike all the other midwives, Nail Helpin had spent six months working with the conventionally trained midwives in the clinic at Amberita. I think this may have been why she was more concerned about antenatal care although, like the other midwives, she said that women would come to her only when they felt in need. Nevertheless, she said she liked women to come to her for massage before the birth, and she also said that women needed to eat well. She had a pair of forceps and surgical scissors which she had bought from the hospital, and these she used for pulling out the placenta and cutting the umbilical cord respectively; she had been taught how to use and sterilize them by the hospital. Despite this training she still retained all her traditional ideas and said she buried the placenta with a little bit of kerosene to make sure the baby didn't cry at night. Like the other midwives, she did not ask for a specific fee: "I don't ask for anything from my clients whatsoever. Whatever they give I'll accept, not like the hospital midwife who demands money even if they are poor. If I did demand money I know that Nenek would come to me in a dream and tell me to help the person who needs it and just to accept whatever they give. So that's what I do."

With all the talk of dreams and the spirituality necessary to become a midwife, Uli injected a certain note of humour when she told us about the dream she'd had in which the "dream woman" had told her that she was *not* the right sort of person to do this work: "When I was younger, about twenty-five I suppose, one of my friends had this dream when the first medicine woman came to her and told her to become a midwife. Apparently she also told her that she didn't choose me because I am very ambitious and not fit for the job. I must say I was really relieved, as then I didn't have to worry about being good and helpful!" Uli also enlightened me about some ceremonies that are still carried out by pregnant women, one of them during the eighth or ninth month of the first pregnancy: "Close relatives come to visit the couple and they have a small party. The couple sit together and the family bring fish to them; then they take a Batak scarf and put it round both their necks and wish them a safe delivery." After the baby is born there is a party at which relatives bring presents, although often nowadays this is in the form of money. This is done only for the first child, not for the others.

Perhaps the midwife I enjoyed meeting the most was Selimatali, a lovely wizened old lady of seventy-five who had helped Uli with her last birth. Looking as if each had a cheek full of boiled sweets – but in fact it was betel nut – they settled down with Letchimi and myself for what they obviously thought would be a comfortable chat in the afternoon. Selimatali was still working as a midwife, and only the previous month she had carried out her first breech delivery. She showed me in detail how she did this, with the woman squatting, and how she caught hold of the legs and carefully drew them up and then, putting her fingers on the baby's jaw, carefully eased the head out. It seemed to me very similar to the technique which I'd seen written up in the textbooks, but when I asked her how she knew what to do she replied, "The spirit showed me." Moreover, with her spirit's help she was confident that she would be able to deal with any sort of delivery, and that nothing would go wrong. She did feel, however, that this birth was extremely uncommon: "If she had come to see me I would have massaged the baby so that it was in the right position to be born in the normal way."

After her husband's death at the hands of the Japanese when she was in her forties, Selimatali had the dream which set her on the road to being a midwife: "I dreamt that Boru Selalehi came from the lake and told me to help pregnant women with their births. But I have always liked to help people, and maybe that is why I had the dream. She said she would help to strengthen my hands and would always be around to help me during birth. I don't do any other general medicine, as she doesn't instruct me. When I am going to deliver a baby, just before going to the house I will sit and pray and ask for the spirit's help. Then when I leave my house the spirit will come with me; I can't see her, but I know she is there helping me. That is why I can tell just by feeling when the baby will be born, and that everything will be all right."

To help women during labour, Selimatali gave them betel leaf with pepper and salt to chew. This probably has a mild painkilling effect, but from her point of view it makes the body hot and means that the woman will give birth more easily. At the same time she massaged the stomach to give the woman the energy to push out the baby: "After the baby is born and the placenta is delivered, I cut the umbilical cord with a piece of bamboo. I put the placenta in a bag with some kerosene and throw it into the lake, but I know that some people like to keep it and bury it."

With the opening of the hospital in Amberita and the partial success of the government's birth control programme, Selimatali now finds that she is not so busy as she used to be: "Sometimes I used to manage three or four births in a day, but now with the hospital midwife I do not have so many. Now I do about one or two a year." Although she didn't request any specific payment, this too had changed: "I don't charge people; it's up to them how much they pay. I used to get six cups of rice for a delivery, but now they pay with money, as much as they can afford." Although the hospital midwife had tried to persuade Selimatali to spend some time in the hospital, she had refused to go: "The hospital midwife called on me as she wanted me to learn their ways, but I refused to go because Boru Selalehi didn't give me permission to do so. She said I needn't go to the hospital and learn their ways because she would continue to teach me and help me in everything I do. She gave me confidence and told me not to be frightened because she is there to help."

The thing I remember most about Selimatali is the tremendous confidence she had in her spirit, which permeated everything she did: "Everything goes well because it is not me doing it but Boru Selalehi. I am now seventy-five years of age, but I will still help anyone who calls me because I have the spirit to help me."

8

A TRADITION OF CARE:
TRADITONAL MIDWIFERY
AMONGST THE MINANGKABAU

DURING THE fourteen-hour journey from Lake Toba to
Bukittinggi there had been plenty of time for me to sample the
delights of Sumatran roads and Sumatran drivers once again.
This time we had come the easy way, on a tourist bus which
had to stop only twice for repairs and with a driver who was
less mad than some. Even so, by the time I arrived I felt as if I
had come from one end of Sumatra to the other. In fact I had
traversed only a third of the island – to those lands in the west
of Sumatra where for centuries the Minangkabau people have
made their home.

According to tradition, the Minangkabau kingdom was
founded by Alexander the Great and established by Hindu
colonists during the seventh century. The name of the
Minangkabau first appeared during the fourteenth century
in a list of lands and districts which owed tribute to the Javanese
kingdom of Madjapahit. From earliest times, however, the
Minangkabau have moved from here to other districts, in
particular to Negeri Sembilan in Malaysia as well as other
parts of Indonesia. The tradition of "going *marantau*", leaving
the homelands to make their fortunes elsewhere, is very well
established and even today is a part of Minangkabau culture.
Young men go to seek their fortune in other far-flung islands
of Indonesia, or even abroad. They take their traditions and

111

establish them in foreign lands, but always keep their connections with the West Sumatran homeland. At the moment there are about two and a half million Minangkabau, 85 per cent of whom live in West Sumatra.

There are several stories about how the Minangkabau got their name, but the one I heard the most often and seemed to be liked the best by the Minangkabau themselves is as follows: "Once, a long time ago, the Javanese came with a great army to conquer our land, but they couldn't. In the end the chiefs decided to settle the issue with a fight between two karabau [or water buffalo]. The Javanese chose their largest and most splendid animal, but the Minangkabau chose a calf which they starved for ten days. On the day of the fight the Minangkabau bound sharp iron points to the calf's horns. The starving calf, in attempting to get milk from the other buffalo, gored it to death, so that the Minangkabau were the victors. To commemorate this event they called their land Minang Kabau, which means the conquering buffalo."

This tale was always told to me with great energy and pride, demonstrating as it did not only the cunning of the Minangkabau (of which they are very proud) but also the strong connection they feel with the water buffalo. Shamsul Aziz is a Minangkabau historian, and he had no doubts about the reasons for this strong and sentimental connection: "In the old days the buffalo was essential for our society. It ploughed the fields and we ate the meat and drank the milk it provided. I think that we honoured the buffalo in our name because in many ways the life of the people depended, and does still depend, on it."

In a place like Bukittinggi there are always groups of guides hanging around the hotels looking for visitors who want to be taken out to see the sights. This was how we met Ad, who at first found it difficult to understand why we didn't want to do the normal tourist-type things. Once he realized that we had different interests, he asked us if we would like to visit his village and talk to the midwife who had delivered him. This was obviously rather a different sort of excursion to what he normally provided, but it sounded exactly right for me. Next day, in the unaccustomed luxury of an air-conditioned bus, we drove through the undulating countryside to Ad's village. On all sides the slopes were divided into neat terraces where men and women with their water buffaloes ploughed, planted and harvested the fields, all of which were at different stages in the rice-growing process. Ad had spent a year with an American family and as a result spoke to us about the country and its people with a most endearing mixed American-Indonesian accent.

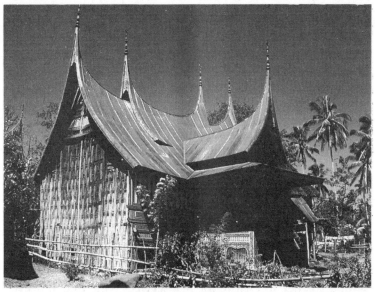

A typical Minangkabau house

Ad's village was up a narrow lane which, with its banks and hedges, reminded me very much of an English village somewhere in Cornwall. The village houses all seemed to be set in higgledy-piggledy fashion, and I couldn't see any with the traditional roof, which has curled points to represent the horns of the water buffalo. Most were ordinary square wooden houses set on short stilts and, like the house of Bie Dara, the midwife, had a small enclosed garden in which grew a profusion of tropical flowers and fruit. She responded to our unforeseen intrusion with marvellous hospitality, and as we all sat down together in her front room I felt more like an old friend than a visitor she had never seen before. Usually the people I talk to are very friendly but even so, as I'm not able to spend much time with them, there is still an element of reserve on both sides. Here there was no feeling of this at all – mainly, I think, because we were accepted as Ad's friends and welcomed as equals on that basis. As we talked I could see that Ad was extremely amused and I think rather surprised that something which to him was so commonplace should provide us with so much pleasure.

Like all the Minangkabau midwives I spoke to, Bie Dara had served a long apprenticeship: "I learnt the massage and everything from my grandfather, Tan Bendarao. He was also the midwife or, as they call it here, *inat pagi*. *Pagi* means baby and *inat* means the man or woman who does the delivery, and in Bahasa Indonesia we translate it as the grandmother of the child." Bie Dara then explained that becoming a midwife depended not only on the practical skills which she had to learn but also on whether she had the right motivation and spiritual qualities: "I became a midwife because I had the urge to do so, I wanted to help people. The most important thing is to want to help and to be able to pray to God for that help. That is why my grandfather also had to show me how to do the *jampi* [prayers] as well." As her main motive in doing the work was to help everyone, she said it would be wrong for her to charge for her services. She did, however, receive a traditional gift called *saripati*, which means "a gift for the midwife" – this could be in kind, chickens or rice, or occasionally money. It was also very important that Bie Dara had the right personal qualities, as these might be passed on to the babies she delivered: "Sometimes I am asked to participate in the river ceremony [when the baby has its first bath, seven days after birth], and if I do, the character of the midwife is thought to be passed on to the child." This was considered a very important responsibility.

Bie Dara had a strong religious orientation in her work: "We believe that whatever medicine I use, it's not so much the medicine that cures the person but the prayers. The medicine

is just a vehicle; it is God who really helps you to get better."
She described a medicine she gave for fever, but cautioned:
"The medicine is just a procedure to ask for help; in other
words, I am just an agent. I make the medicine and ask for
God's help, and He blesses it so that the person gets well."
Although Bie Dara had been taught practical skills, these were
always in the context of a religious focus: "I learnt what to do
by seeing the things my grandfather did, but we also believe
that you have to know the right prayers so that God will
help. That is our philosophy of learning here; you have to
understand the whole situation."

The Minangkabau are Muslim and have been so for many
hundreds of years, since the faith first arrived some time
between the fourteenth and sixteenth centuries. By the eighteenth century, however, there were many who had not
converted, and it was only at the beginning of the nineteenth
century, when imams resorted to force, killing and enslaving,
that the majority of the population became Muslim. Their
original faith was Hindu, and although nowadays all the
Minangkabau profess to be Muslims, remnants of this old
faith can still be found. They have kept some of their
pre-Islamic customs, one of the most important being the
way in which families are traced through the female rather
than the male line. Bie Dara talked a lot about *jampi*,
incantations or prayers, but was unwilling to divulge much
about them. Undoubtedly some were Muslim prayers, but
I wondered if there were also prayers and incantations from
pre-Muslim times.

Exploring Minangkabau beliefs shows that Islamic ideas
are paramount, although there are elements of paganism
and Hinduism. It is believed that there are seven heavens
– although at face value this seems to be a Hindu belief, it
also matches in with Islamic ideas which say that Mohammed
climbed to the seventh heaven. While Allah is thought to be
the Creator and supreme being, there are countless other
good and bad spirits which work for good and evil and can
be contacted and used. The soul is thought to be a tripartite
entity, the most important part being *njawa*, which means

"life-bearer" or "life principle". This is thought of as the "real soul", which leaves the body at death. *Sumangat* is the life force or consciousness, which is the part of the soul most involved with health. *Sumangat* can leave the body during dreams, and this can be effected voluntarily by some people. It leaves involuntarily during illness, which can be brought on by fright, anxiety or because of evil spirits. To cure illness one has to get the *sumangat* to return, as if it doesn't it will weaken the *njawa* so much that it will leave and the person will die. The Minangkabau believe that animals and plants, as well as humans, have souls, and that rice has the same sort of soul as humans. For this reason they have elaborate rice ceremonies, the aim of which is to protect the soul of the rice so that the whole harvest will be good. A plant is taken out of the field for this ritual, and it is believed that the rice soul is concentrated in this plant. The rice ritual is then enacted to summon the highest good of the rice crop; the rice soul concentrated in this plant attracts the souls of all the other plants and ensures a good crop.

Bie Dara thought that the most useful thing she did for mothers was massage: "The most important thing in childbirth is how the child lies inside the mother, and I massage during pregnancy to make sure it is in the right position. I also give herbal medicine to make the mother strong – I say prayers over this, of course." Massage was given any time antenatally, depending on when the woman wanted it: "It can be in the first month or any month. Whenever she feels like it."

She then explained some of the things a woman should do to ensure an easy birth: "When a woman is pregnant she shouldn't sit in a door entrance or gateway because the baby may find it difficult to get out. If she goes down to the river to bathe, she mustn't come back until she's finished; if she's forgotten something she shouldn't come back to the house for it, as this could delay the delivery. Also when a pregnant mother wants anything to eat, the family will get it for her, otherwise, after the baby is born, it will have a lot of saliva coming out of its mouth. The pregnant lady shouldn't see bad things happening; also she shouldn't speak badly about other people. In fact, women who are not pregnant shouldn't speak badly about others, but it's particularly important for women who are pregnant, as this could have a bad effect on the baby. During the pregnancy she should eat a lot of fried eel, since this is shiny and slippery and will help the baby to slip out easily."

It is tempting to see these ideas as no more than superstition: what causal connection can there possibly be between sitting in a doorway and a difficult birth? I do wonder, however, if by having her attention brought to her body in this way, and by symbolically "clearing the way" for the baby to come out easily, a woman is in fact helped physically to give birth. After all, there are plenty of documented cases where various forms of mental imagery have been used to help cure physical illness such as cancer. Is this not another form of imagery, and why shouldn't it work just as well?

In Bie Dara's experience, birth normally took about half to one hour, and I think she was just talking about the second stage when the baby is pushed out. She acknowledged that the woman might be in labour before this, but as far as she was concerned this time when the baby was pushed out was the most crucial part of the labour. The woman took whatever position was most comfortable to do this: "Sometimes they squat, sometimes they lie down – she can do it whatever way is comfortable." On the whole, Bie Dara said she did not have many problem births, but where there was a delay she thought this was often because there were problems between the mother and her family, the most important of these relationships being the one between the pregnant woman and her own mother. If there was delay, the labouring woman would ask forgiveness from her mother for any sins she had committed against her. Bie Dara would then massage the woman, and the baby would be born. If this didn't work, other members of the family would be brought so that the woman could ask for forgiveness from them as well. In Bie Dara's experience this usually worked, and the baby was born with no further delay.

Once the baby was born, Bie Dara cut the umbilical cord

a piece of bamboo. She then explained how important it was to bury the placenta in the right place: "If you want the child to stay near home, you bury the placenta under the front step of the house; but if you want the child to go and make his fortune away, you bury the placenta away from the house." After birth Bie Dara gave the mother herbal remedies and as much massage as she wanted until she was able to resume normal life and work. This midwife obviously loved her work and felt that there was much more she could have told me. As I left she cheerfully said "There are all sorts of things I could teach you if you came and stayed here with me for a while." Oh that I could!

Ad had asked Bie Dara about another midwife who lived in a village nearby. In contrast to Ad's village this one had a very open aspect, with houses scattered over a large area of land. Some of them were of the traditional kind, with roofs that had a pair or more of points which are said to represent the horns of their beloved buffalo, although another theory says that they represent the type of small boat that the original inhabitants used to get to this land. A Minangkabau traditional family house can be quite large, rectangular in shape and built on piles, the roof projecting over a long front balcony. Stone steps lead up to the front room, the main room of the house, in which there is a fireplace and where all family discussions will take place. There are usually various small rooms behind this large one, and in the past a single family home could house seventy or eighty people, all descended from the same ancestral mother. Despite the greater affluence there are now fewer of these houses, as Ad explained: "It is now so expensive to build a horn-shaped roof, and an ordinary roof is much cheaper. Only the rich can afford to do it now; the poor have ordinary houses."

In addition to the houses this village also had rice granaries, a *balai* or communal house, and a mosque in front of which was the water supply. This was an important meeting place for villagers (especially the women) who came to wash and collect water, as well as being the religious centre of the village. Like most villages this one also had a *tabua*, a large ceremonial drum which used to be used as a warning and signal for meetings but is now used mainly during Ramadan to signal the beginning and end of the fast each day. Ad told me that the *balai* is used by the young boys of the village for sleeping after they reach the age of about eight. He didn't have to do this as his parents had a house sufficiently large for the boys and girls to be separated. This is often the case nowadays, although in some villages the tradition of the boys sleeping in the *balai* continues.

Finding the midwife took some time, as there were many houses fairly far apart and Ad collected quite a following of children and others as he walked around looking for her. Eventually we found her, a very young-looking woman (aged about forty-nine) who cheerfully said she'd be delighted to talk to us. We sat in her small hut surrounded by a huge crowd of interested people who quietly listened as we talked. Nurleta had been practising on her own for only one year, since her mother had died, but was very aware of the age-old family tradition of her work: "I learnt the midwifery work from my mother and she learnt it from her mother and it goes back a long way. Normally it is passed on from mother to daughter and it goes on from generation to generation, so when a mother dies her daughter will take over. While my mother was alive I only helped her to do the deliveries, and I learnt by watching what she was doing. I started learning the prayers when I was about twelve or thirteen years old." As the only woman left in her family, Nurleta felt she had certain responsibilities: "Since my sister died having her last child [in the hospital] I am the only woman left in my family to carry on these traditions and later pass them on to my daughters. I like being a midwife and I also help those who have other problems that can be eased with massage – strains and things like that."

Like Bie Dara, Nurleta thought it was important that pregnant women came to her antenatally for massage, although always in the context of what they thought they needed: "I like women to come to me for massage when they are about four months pregnant, not before. How many times they have the massage depends on the woman, but if the baby is in the wrong position I can massage it into the right place ready for birth." In order that women should have an easy birth Nurleta had a list, similar to Bie Dara's, of symbolic things which pregnant women should and shouldn't do.

Once labour starts, Nurleta would be called to the woman's house, where she said the first thing she would do would be to make the mother a drink out of special leaves and herbs over which she would chant some prayers. The woman would then drink from this three times, the rest would be put on her stomach, and Nurleta would massage it in. For the rest of the labour Nurleta would massage to help the labouring woman through the pains. In Nurleta's experience birth rarely took more than three hours and was much more likely to only take half an hour or so, but if the baby was delayed she would give the mother some special herbal medicine. For a breech birth she felt there was no need to do anything special: "If the feet come out first I don't do anything except massage very gently. It takes a bit longer, but after a while the baby comes out safely. When the baby comes out I cut the umbilical cord with a piece of bamboo and then throw away the placenta in the river. In this village we all like the children to leave home, as only if they go out can they learn more things and be successful. We leave the umbilical cord on the baby's stomach to dry up and fall off, and then we throw that away as well." After the birth Nurleta ties up the mother's stomach with a piece of cloth or a sarong after giving some more massage.

Nurleta then told me in more detail about the first bath in the river, which in this village was still an important ritual for the baby: "After about nine days, after the umbilical cord has fallen off, we take the baby for its first bath in the river. In this village the father usually takes the baby to the river, but in some places the mother or the midwife will do so. When they get down to the river, the religious man will cut off a few hairs (twenty-one or seven or something like that) and the baby will be named. When they get back to the house prayers will be said, and then everyone will have a small feast."

Later on, in Bukittinggi, I talked to Shamsul Aziz in some detail about the matrilineal nature of Minangkabau society which I had heard about in passing from both the midwives I'd talked to. Minangkabau men and women trace their lineage and obtain their inheritance through the women rather than the men, with the clan being headed by the oldest woman of the group. Two sorts of possessions are recognized: those that belong to the clan, called *harto pusako*, which include all the things that sustain life (rice fields, land, gold/silver, weapons and karabau) and those that are individually owned, usually money and possessions that a person has amassed during a lifetime. Things which belong to the clan cannot be sold except in exceptional circumstances, when every member of the clan must agree to it; they can be passed only to other females in the clan. Individual wealth may be distributed in any way the individual likes, but often some of it will be given to the clan to become clan property. In the past land was divided into *tanah mati* (dead or uncultivated land), which belonged to all, and *tanah hidui* (alive or cultivated land), which belonged to individual families. This latter belonged to the family of the original cultivator of the land, but no family was allowed to have more land than they needed for their support. There were therefore no very large estates owned by families who were unable to do all the work themselves. The family title was always held and inherited by women.

The leader of the clan, however, is a man, usually the brother of the eldest woman in the clan. As Shamsul Aziz explained, "I am the chief of my family, as my elder sister is the oldest woman in my clan, which is called the Karo. When anyone in the family wants to get married or if they have problems, like not having enough money, they will come and see me and we will talk about it and discuss how the problem can be solved." This happened despite the fact that individuals within the Karo clan were now very far-flung in different parts of Indonesia: "There are about twenty families in my clan, and most of them don't live in the village any more. Some of them are in Jakarta and different parts of Indonesia, but we all keep in touch about what is happening

121

to all of us. Of course my son and two daughters belong to my wife's clan."

This arrangement meant that in the past woman in Minangkabau society had a considerable amount of power. This was seen in the marriages, where a man did not gain possession of a wife on marriage and had no rights over her except that she was expected to be faithful. For the woman, the man was expected to visit her regularly, and if he did not this was sufficient grounds for divorce. The first marriage might be arranged by the family, but if this did not work out the couple were then free to marry again, whomever they chose. It was not unknown for women to have had six husbands by the time they were twenty or so. The children were brought up by the female members of the family, and on divorce would live in the family house of their mother. The men were not usually involved with decisions about the children, as these were seen as a female concern.

On marriage a man would join his wife's family, but as a new member of the family had to be very careful about relationships with his in-laws: "When a man becomes a new member of his wife's family he mustn't jump directly into all the problems. He must listen to what everybody else says before putting his point of view, and he must wait until he's asked before making suggestions and that sort of thing. This is how he must live in his new family." Shamsul thought that with the overall changes in society and nuclear families now living more individual lives, children were guided more by their father than by their mother. Society might have changed and clans were more dispersed, but there was still a very strong link between members, and much of the customary *adat*, especially that of inheritance, was still being adhered to. This was helped by the very large number of Minangkabau associations, not only in Indonesia but also as far a way as California, which allowed people to keep in touch and knowledge of what was happening with individual clan members to be disseminated far and wide.

Amongst the Minangkabau there is considerable pride in their tradition of democracy. The smallest unit of independent government is the clan, where issues are discussed and decided within each family. Their views are put to the village *penghulus* (leaders) who form the village council to make decisions about village affairs and communal property. Decisions are mad according to native *adat* and Muslim law, but all decisions must be made with a unanimous vote and be acceptable to the families which the *penghulus* represent. Access to office is a matter of inheritance, but the family must feel that the person has the right qualifications, and if he does not fulfil his obligations in a way that is satisfactory to the family they have no compunction about replacing him. While the Minangkabau still have a king and noble families, they have no role or influence in the wider government of Minangkabau society.

Maridiana lived in another village some way from Bukitt-inggi, and when I met her I just could not believe that she was seventy-five years old. Her skin had a lovely bloom, with no wrinkles, and she moved with both grace and energy as she invited us into her spotless house. She told me that she took special herbs every day to achieve this, and that was how she was able to continue helping with the birth of up to seventy-five babies each year: "I learnt about all the traditional medicine from my father, who was a *dukun*; he taught me how to *jampi*, how to prepare the herbs, how to massage, and all that sort of thing." A *dukun* amongst the Minangkabau can be male or female, and I was interested to hear of so many midwives who had learnt their craft from a male, although I never came across a modern male practitioner.

Many *dunkuns* have a specialism such as massage, herbal remedies or circumcision, but as well as this practical skill they are also able to deal with evil spirits through prayer and the use of magic. They are seers rather than shamans, as the spirits do not actually enter them, although they are able to contact and manipulate them. Some *dukuns*, with the help of friendly spirits, go to the land of the spirits to bring back lost souls who may have either wandered or been abstracted. Not all do this, however, and *dukuns* are respected for whatever specialism they possess. *Maridiana*, however, had also learnt from other sources and was able

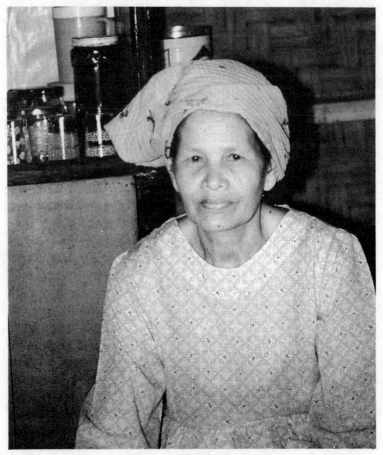

Maridiana, a Minangkabau midwife

to integrate a variety of different viewpoints with no apparent difficulty: "I also learnt from a German doctor who was here in the fifties and I often accompanied him when he went out to do deliveries. I've been doing this work now for about thirty years." In addition to midwifery, Maridiana knew about medicines for a wide range of different illnesses. She was also hoping that her knowledge would be passed on within the family: "My daughter is just starting to learn, and my sister has already learnt all the massage. This way the knowledge will be passed on from generation to generation."

Maridiana would go to the woman's house when she was in labour: "First I'll massage her head, then her forehead, and then her hips. And then, when I see the signs that the baby is going to come out, I will ask her to lie down and I give her a special herbal drink so that the baby will come out smoothly and nothing will go wrong." The majority of women whom she had helped to give birth would already have come to her for massage: "Most of the women here come to me when they are in their second month of pregnancy. Then they come maybe once or twice a week for a massage – it really depends on them: whether they feel like it or whether they think they need it." Even when women went to the hospital for checkups they still came to her for massage, both before and after the birth. In her experience birth took about half an hour, but it could delay for as long as twenty-four hours and in this case she would *jampi* and massage, which she said, in her experience, always worked very well.

After birth she used scissors to cut the umbilical cord, after which she threw the placenta away. She had a different version of what used to be done with the placenta, and why: "They used to say that if you threw the placenta away the baby would cry day and night for the first seven days of its life, but if you buried it this would ensure that the baby wouldn't cry. But before I throw it away I always say the *jampi* so that nothing goes wrong. I learnt this from my father." Maridiana remembered a time when "the fire treatment" (the woman sitting near or lying over a fire) was more common after birth, but said that she didn't use it nowadays. Instead she filled a bottle with hot water, wrapped it in a cloth and tied it round the woman's stomach. Afterwards she did what sounded like a fairly crude form of binding to help the woman regain her shape: "I take a small towel, fold it into a pad and put it on her stomach, pushing it up to put the womb back into place. I then bind it there with a piece of cloth." She also massaged for up to three months after the birth, again depending on what the new mother felt she wanted and needed.

Many of Maridiana's clients went to the hospital for check-ups, if not for the birth, but even if they did not give birth with her she would do the massage for them before and afterwards. She said there was no compulsion from the hospital midwife to give birth in the hospital, and had no idea how many women were now deciding to do so. The hospital had, however, been found wanting as far as family planning services were concerned, and Maridiana found herself giving more help in this field than previously: "The Indonesian government has gone all out for family planning and a lot of people have started coming to me for birth control. If you go to the hospital they give you pills or injections, but a lot of people don't like them because they have side-effects; so they come to me. What I do is to massage for forty days, pushing up the womb as I do so. On the fortieth day I give her this special medicine to drink; I call it *tahan nya* [which literally means 'control it'] and after that she won't have any more children."

I enjoyed talking to Maridiana immensely. She was so welcoming and, like Bie Dara, said that if I wanted to learn more I could come and stay with her and she would teach me.

The last Minangkabau midwife I talked to was Millun, who at the age of eighty-five was even older, but with loads of energy and a very mischievous smile. She began by telling me proudly that she still had all her teeth, explaining that she had accomplished this because all her life she had chewed sirih and gambir. She said she had been doing midwifery for fifty years, but carried out only the practical, not the magical, aspects of it: "I give them herbal medicine, but I don't *jampi*. I just believe in God and ask Him to help. Oh no! I don't have any special prayers, I just pray to God to help me so that nothing goes wrong." Like all the other midwives Millun started massaging when the woman was about four months pregnant, and did as little or as much as she wanted.

When giving birth, Millun said, the woman would almost invariably squat. After tying the umbilical cord with cotton, Millun then cut it with a bamboo splinter: "I don't throw the placenta away, I just bury it. There's no particular reason and I don't think it affects the baby at all, whatever you do. I just don't like to throw it away, that's all." After the birth she said she massaged the mother for about half an hour: "Then I tie up the stomach with a cotton belt and give her a drink made of banana and papaya root. That's all we do these days, although years ago I used to do the fire treatment, but nowadays no one wants it."

Millun felt that she provided an important service, mainly to the poorer people in her village: "The rich people who have a lot of money, they go to the hospital and give birth there, but the poor come to me. I don't charge a certain amount like the hospital – whatever they can afford to pay me I accept, and if they can't afford anything, that's also something I accept." The hospital midwife visited the village, and for the first time since I had been in this area I detected a certain amount of tension between traditional and more conventional medical practitioners: "The hospital midwife did visit the village, but she wouldn't talk to me or teach me how to do things. After that I decided that I didn't want to be taught because after all this time I know what I'm doing." Whatever the hospital did, however, she still felt that there would be people who needed her: "The number of people coming to me is smaller than it used to be because a lot now go to the hospital. I still help with the delivery for the people who still need me."

As with so many of the midwives I talked to, I felt a tremendous affinity with Millun and a respect for what she was doing. When I left she gave me a big hug and said I was welcome to come and see her again whenever I felt like it.

9

A SIMPLE AFFAIR: BIRTH AMONGST THE TORAJA

THE NAME "Toraja" means "men of the mountains" and was given to the people who lived in the central highlands of Sulawesi by the lowland dwellers of this island. During the Dutch rule of Indonesia this peculiarly shaped island was called Celebes, and its main town, Makassar, was for many years an important centre of the spice trade. To get there from Sumatra had taken us a long three days by boat.

Buses now run regularly from Ujung Pandang (the name with which Makassar was rechristened) to Rantepao, the centre of the Torajan homelands in the mountains. Unlike Sumatran buses they were not, on the whole, full to overflowing, but as they rushed along the narrow roads with squealing of brakes and roaring of engines, spitting out black exhaust, they reminded me of raging elephants. The driver of our bus was erratic and fast, braking heavily as he swung it from side to side, using its horn and its bulk to overwhelm everything else stupid or unlucky enough to get in his way.

The land around Ujung Pandang is very flat and productive. Rice fields stretched as far as the eye could see in all directions with, every so often, odd houses rearing up in their midst on tall stilts. As we climbed up into the mountains, the bus careering round the hairpin bends with ever-increasing abandon, the flat valleys gave way to the most breathtaking mountain scenery. We drove through long valleys, their sides terraced with rice fields which gradually dissolved into clumps of trees which themselves then dissolved into bare and fantastically shaped craggy mountain tops. The closer we got to Rantepao, the more Torajan houses we saw, their huge roofs sweeping up to the sky at both ends. They are large and imposing, yet when I came to walk around the Torajan countryside I was surprised how these huge, decorated houses blended in so well. It was very easy just to walk past without noticing. Part of it may have been my lack of attention, of course, but I also felt that the houses were built to harmonize with their surroundings, not to dominate the landscape.

Rantepao is the last stop for all the ordinary buses and has the air of a frontier town. In its midst is a huge expanse of scruffy-looking land which serves as the market square every sixth day of the Toraja week. On market day it becomes a sea of colour, with people squatting down by their mats selling their wares. There are rows of little shops which, although catering for the recent influx of tourists, also sell the more mundane necessities of life. Almost as soon as we arrived we saw one of the people from the surrounding villages walking into the town carrying several long bamboo pipes of *tuak*, the local alcoholic brew. This, a fermented sap collected from palm trees, is extremely popular. We watched as someone tried a few drops, this being done with a small "spoon" made of twisted palm leaf. As he was apparently happy with the taste, he bought the whole pipeful.

The Toraja are often described as being similar to the Bataks, and it is true that they did have a very fierce reputation for cannibalism and headhunting. Living in scattered villages which were difficult to reach, they maintained their mountain stronghold against all attacks from the coastal people until they were pacified by the Dutch in 1907. At this time, the Toraja were led by the legendary Pong Tilsu, who managed the almost impossible task of bringing the scattered Toraja together to fight for their group as a whole. In the end, however, he was defeated by the Dutch, who set up a system of government and administration for the whole of Tana Toraja and insisted that villages were moved to the valleys, where they were more accessible. They abolished headhunting and slavery, the latter being one of the main ways, together with the trade in coffee, in which the Torajan upper class had created and maintained their wealth. Not surprisingly there was considerable resistance to these changes, although today older Torajans will grudgingly admit that the Dutch rule did bring peace and was far superior to that of the Japanese during World War II.

A few days after our arrival we were driving out of Rantepao with Marthen, who had agreed to take us to see the traditional midwife in his village. Once out of Rantepao there was no question of going quickly as the jeep bumped painfully along over the patches and potholes of which the road was made. We came at the time of a bumper rice harvest and people were busily harvesting, a row of men and women working patiently in a line through the rice, cutting each stalk individually and tying them into bunches. This laborious method is used so that the rice will not be scared by the knife and will therefore produce a good harvest the following year. In the middle of each rice field is a large hole which is permanently filled with water and is for the fish which are now an important part of the Toraja diet. Looking at the terraced fields which went up in ever-decreasing size to almost the tops of the mountains, and the water system which supported them, it was difficult to imagine that they had been here for less than a hundred years. Originally the Toraja grew crops by the slash and burn method, together with hunting, gathering and grazing buffalo herds on the hillside. Even before the Dutch arrived land was in short supply, and the once forested hills had become denuded. With the support of the Dutch the Toraja began growing wet rice, and the terraces now look as if they have been there for ever.

When we arrived at Marthen's village I was pleased to see that it was one of the older kind, consisting of a row of traditional houses opposite which was a row of rice barns.

There is a much-disputed legend that the design of the houses reflects an ancient memory of the ships in which the first Toraja arrived in Sulawesi. Each house is elevated on piles and dominated by a roof which sweeps up high at each end and does put one in mind of the prow of a ship. The roof is covered with short pieces of bamboo slotted together; these are even more durable then the sheets of corrugated iron that are now used by many people. The latter, however, are often preferred, not only for their cheapness, but because they are lighter and easier to work with.

Marthen showed us his family house, which was one of the larger ones, made with no nails and decorated with traditional geometric and pictorial motifs in different shades of orange and brown. It was only later, when I watched someone painting these designs for a funeral, that I realized they were all done entirely freehand. On a pole which stretched from the top of the roof at the front to the ground were fixed a very large number of buffalo horns, showing how many buffalo had been killed for various family death ceremonies. Inside the house it was very dark, with a central room which was used for cooking and eating. There were bedrooms at each end, the one on the south side being used to keep the dead bodies in before the death feast and the one on the north side being used by the family when it stayed there. The family now lived in Rantepao and returned to this house only for family festivals like the death ceremony.

It was not long before Martha Billam arrived, a vibrant woman in her fifties or sixties with betel-stained teeth and a mobile and expressive face. Apparently she was very well known for her midwifery skills, not only in the village where she lived but in other villages where she might be asked to go and help if a woman seemed to be in exceptional difficulty. She had been taught how to be a midwife by her mother: "After my mother died she came to me in a dream and gave me some grass, and then I knew I could start doing the midwife's work. It was about twenty years ago and I've been doing it ever since then." The main technique that Martha used to help women both during pregnancy and birth was massage:

"I don't have any special prayers or anything like that. I can't even read or write; I only believe in God and do the massage." Unlike the Batak midwives, who continued to keep in touch with their spiritual helper, Martha said that after this initial visit from her mother in a dream she no longer had contact with her, although she believed that her mother was still alive in the spirit world.

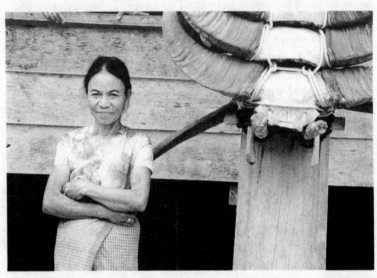

Martha standing by her house, on which were the horns of many buffalo killed for death celebrations

Women usually started coming to see Martha early on in pregnancy: "Once I massage I can tell whether the woman is pregnant or not, and also how many months pregnant she is. The women first come to me when they are three months pregnant, then they may come again at seven months and again just before they give birth. But whenever they need me to do the massage I'll go; whatever the time of the day or night." Martha thought that much of the pain in childbirth was induced through fear: "The birth can take any time, but often it is only half or one hour, not often more than three hours. But sometimes a woman will say, 'It hurts, it hurts' just because she is scared, and that makes the pain feel worse. I do some massage and this helps her to feel calmer, and the pain lessens. I can tell when the baby will be born just by feeling. Sometimes a woman will have pains and think that the baby will be born soon, but if I touch her I can tell that it won't come until next week, and I'm usually right."

After the baby was born, Martha cut the umbilical cord with bamboo after first boiling it to ensure that the cut wouldn't make the baby itch. She said that normally she buried the placenta, but the only reason she had for doing this was because it was "the Toraja way" – the way it had always been done unless the mother had experienced problem births: "If a woman has had several babies that have died, we'll hang the cord and placenta on a palm tree. No one should drink the wine from that tree. No, I don't know why we do it, but it will help her present baby to live." Martha also believed that if the umbilical cord was short, the baby would be sickly, but if it was long, the baby would be healthy.

When I asked her if she ever did any binding of the stomach for women after birth, she hooted with laughter: "Usually it's only the town women who ask for that. We village women don't need it as we're healthy and our stomachs go back flat without all that binding." After birth Martha said she would massage only if the mother needed it, and many didn't. As far as she knew there were no special birth ceremonies (apart from Christian baptism) and no special food for a mother to eat or things she should and shouldn't do. Apart from taking things a little easy for a week or two after birth, there was nothing special to mark this event.

On the whole, men did not participate in the birth unless there was some delay in the delivery: "Then the husband will be brought in, wash the back of his feet and give the water to the lady to drink. This is symbolic of washing away all the sins, not only between them but in the rest of the family, which may be delaying the birth." If the baby came out feet first, "I have to help the mother by massaging and helping her to bring out the child. But this very rarely happens because before the baby comes I can feel its position and turn it round the right way." For excess bleeding Martha used two herbal remedies, depending on whether the blood was thick or thin.

Although the village was several miles away from Rantepao, Martha said that more women were now visiting the hospital there: "But if women don't get the right sort of help at the hospital they'll come to me for massage. The hospital is good for some things such as if the woman doesn't have enough blood and things like that." She said that people weren't forced to go to the hospital and it was generally the better off who did so.

In a year Martha delivered about twenty babies, but her time was also taken up treating other physical problems such as fevers and other childhood illnesses as well as helping women who were having difficulties getting pregnant. She wouldn't carry out abortions and said that in any case, in spite of the government's birth control campaign, families around the village still liked to have several children, as it meant there were a lot of people to help with the death ceremony. She didn't charge any particular amount for her services: "It is up to the people I help as to what they give; some give me a sarong or a blouse and some give me money. I will accept anything they like to give me."

As we left the village I noticed someone sitting under one of the rice barns, feeding a water buffalo. "What on earth are they doing that for?" I asked. "Can't the buffalo feed itself?"

Marthen looked at me as if I were a small child who had asked a very obvious question. "The trouble with buffaloes", he began, "is that they are very lazy and if you leave it up to them they won't get very fat. We like to have our buffaloes fat, so someone has to feed it."

To the Toraja the buffalo is a symbol of wealth and therefore status, and I was amused to see Marthen shudder slightly when I asked him if they were used to work the fields. "Oh no! They're far too valuable!" was the reply as he went on to explain how the number of buffalo that a family owns is a measure of its wealth and the number they kill at a ceremony, particularly a death ceremony, is an even better indicator.

The life of a Torajan buffalo is one of indolence; a small boy will spend much of his time looking after it, leading it around to find the most succulent grass and feeding it to make sure that it gets suitably fat. When it is hot the buffalo will be bathed and made to stand under the cool trees while its keeper finds it even more to eat. At the end, of course, the buffalo will be a sacrifice, probably at a death feast, and only then will the Torajans eat the meat, although they will drink the milk (which is thought to have some medicinal value) of the much less valuable female buffalo.

On the way back to Rantepao we stopped to talk to another midwife, Nek Reke, a woman with a seamed face and strong hands who must have been in her seventies. We had to walk across several fields of rice *padi* to get to her house, which seemed to be quite isolated. Nevertheless, as we talked together sitting on a mat in the shade of her home, we gradually became surrounded by an ever-increasing crowd of boisterous children. Chewing betel in a contented way and spitting out the red juice in all directions, she told me how she had learnt the skills of midwifery from her grandmother. She had been doing this work for many years, since she was young, and quite unusually for a Toraja had only a small family of two children – both of whom were grown up.

Women normally first came to her when they were three or four months pregnant: "If a woman has sickness, then it shows that the baby is in the wrong position. I don't give medicine for it, I massage the baby round to the right position and then she feels better. Once a lady can feel the baby move, I start doing the massage regularly and this helps the baby grow well." While giving birth some women would lie down, some would squat and others would kneel. Much to the delight of the crowd, Nek Reke then demonstrated on me what she would do with someone kneeling or squatting to give birth: "I sit behind her and massage and hold her hips, but if a woman gives birth lying down I massage her stomach as the baby comes out." In her experience birth did not usually take very long, although she was talking about the second stage rather than the whole process of labour and birth as it is generally discussed in medical textbooks. In her experience it might take as short a time as five minutes or more usually about an hour or two, although it could be delayed for a day. If the baby was delayed she didn't do anything special apart from massaging and encouraging the mother.

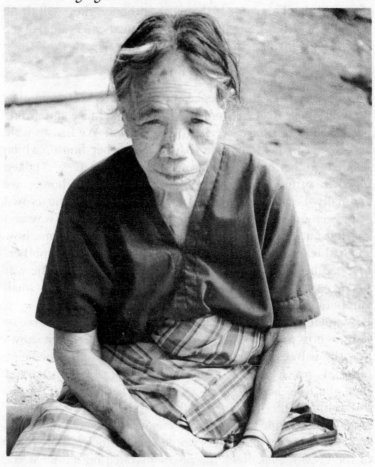

Nek Reke

A Simple Affair: Birth Amongst the Toraja

Once the child was born, she cut the umbilical cord with a piece of bamboo: "If it is old bamboo that has been in the house I just take it and use it, but if it is freshly cut I boil it before doing the cutting so that the wound won't itch. I tie the cord with a piece of string before I cut." She was the only Torajan midwife I came across who had an explanation for burying the placenta: "We bury the placenta and umbilical cord so that when the child grows up they will be very productive in their lives. If you don't bury it the child won't be very fortunate – maybe poor and finding it difficult to earn money." Nek Reke also told me about a belief that if, after being buried, the placenta turns into a stone, the family would become very rich.

Nek Reke did not, on the whole, have many problems with birth and did not think it was particularly dangerous: "Everyone works hard and is very healthy here." For excess bleeding she just asked the woman to lie still afterwards, but she said that this could be quite a good thing and that it was in fact far more dangerous if there was no blood coming out afterwards: "It is healthy if the woman bleeds after the baby is born because that means that all the dirty blood is coming out. If the blood doesn't come out afterwards I have to massage for the blood to come, otherwise it will go thick inside and lead to other problems." She continued her care after the birth, massaging for two or three days afterwards depending on what was needed: "This is to put back the womb in its right position."

She confirmed Martha's assertion that nothing special was done after birth and that women went back to work in a week or so depending on how they felt and the needs of the family. Occasionally Nek Reke was asked to do a stomach binding, but this was not a common request and was usually made by those from the town. One day after the birth of the baby Nek Reke said some families might have a little party. If they were Christians the minister would come in and christen the child; if they were animists the priestly equivalent would do the same thing to give thanks for the safe delivery.

Although Nek Reke lived in what seemed like splendid

isolation in the middle of *padi* fields she was not far away from Rantepao, and she was therefore very aware of the activities of the hospital there. Many of her richer clients came to her for massage and then went on to give birth at the hospital. On several occasions she had actually gone to help with people giving birth there: "It is mainly the poorer people who come to me because they can't afford to go to the hospital. They can just pay me what they can afford or they can even give me rice if they prefer. The rich people come to me for massage and then for the delivery they go to the hospital, although if they have any difficulties they might call for me. I think that those women who give birth with me are healthier than those who go to the hospital, and I think they have healthier babies as well." Whether she thought hospital had a causative effect I couldn't say, although maybe those who thought they were less healthy opted for a hospital delivery. Nek Reke felt that as they didn't use massage in the hospital they couldn't really know what was going on inside the body in quite the same way that she could.

Another midwife I talked to in Rantepao was Indo Katapi. She was very deaf, and interviewing her was a somewhat protracted affair requiring the help of one of the good-natured women at the restaurant which we frequented. Indo Katapi's services were apparently very much in demand and this was just as well, as she was responsible for four grandchildren whom she had started looking after when one of her daughters had died a few years previously. Like most of the other midwives, she had learnt how to do the massage from her mother and said that she had been doing it since she was young, although now she was older and less strong she found it more difficult: "Women come to me from the first month of pregnancy and depending on what they want, I will massage them all through the pregnancy. If they feel pain they'll come to me. I do the massage with oil which has had onion mixed with it." In her experience, which included helping at the births of every one of her twenty-six grandchildren, most women either knelt or squatted to give birth. Although she had experienced delays and difficult births, she did not feel there was any danger in it.

Unlike the other midwives she cut the umbilical cord with scissors rather than bamboo and then buried the placenta which, she said, was a popular thing to do: "Even if people give birth in the hospital they bring back the placenta and umbilical cord and bury them near the house. This is how we Torajans have always done it." After the birth she massaged the woman every day for two or three days, depending on the needs of her client. She said that she had experienced one or two breech births, and these were more difficult than normal births. She massaged the stomach more intensively to help the woman give birth, and it usually took a bit longer. If there were any difficulties with breastfeeding she would massage the breasts to help the milk flow, and she said that eating raw peanuts also helped. Many of Indo Katapi's clients now went to the hospital, but she said they came back to her after the birth for massage.

Apart from helping pregnant women, she also had other clients: "If someone has swollen hands or their bones move a bit I can massage them straight. Also if anyone dislocates a joint I can put it back and I also do massage for various pains, especially stomach pain, and fevers." Despite her own very difficult financial circumstances Indo Katapi did not ask for a fee for her work and, like the others, was willing to accept whatever her clients could afford to pay her. If they could not afford money, however, she said she would ask for rice instead, because she badly needed it to feed her grandchildren. Her eyes really lit up when I gave her some money as a "thank you" for helping me and I hoped she enjoyed spending it, although undoubtedly it would go on necessities for her family.

Talking to these midwives, I was struck at how simple birth seemed to be compared to death which, as we saw when we attended a death ceremony, required protracted and expensive rituals. Just after World War II Harry Wilcox spent six months living in a Toraja village. He commented on how simple birth seemed to be and, as he said, "Birth is not an occasion for fuss." He noticed that women observed few taboos either before or after the birth, although a father was not supposed to leave the house, especially during the hours of darkness, for three days or nights after his wife had given birth. He once came upon a little burial mound close to the house which had a small stockade around it, and was told this was a placenta which had been buried and that the stockade was to keep out evil spirits which, if they got into the placenta, might have power over the baby. I had also noticed that compared with some of the other groups I had visited, Torajan midwives did not seem to have an overt spiritual context in which to work. Even Christian ideas were infrequently mentioned. Their death ceremonies, however, seemed as important and popular as ever, and I wondered why this was so.

I later found an explanation for this in the experiences which the Torajan's underwent as a result of colonization by the Dutch. Precolonially there was no word for "religion" to describe something which was transcendent to the actions required for ordinary living. Human and spiritual action were fused in the concept of *aluk*, which covered a whole range of things: the wisdom of the ancestors, spirits, speeches of the priests, the 7,777 prohibitions which informed daily life, and the proper performance of every prayer and ceremony. Originally it was believed that the world began when the sky descended to the earth in an embrace of love as a result of which three sons were born. Each of these sons was responsible for a different part of the cosmos – below and above earth, as well as earth itself. From these three brothers and their wives came the earth as the Toraja know it as well as the customs necessary to live there successfully.

These higher gods, however, were not of much direct concern to those on earth. Of much more importance were the *deata* and the ancestors who, provided the rituals were properly held, would bestow their blessings on the living.

Ceremonies were divided into "smoke rising" ceremonies, which include all those related to the east side of life – birth, growth and prosperity – and "smoke descending" ceremonies, connected with the west – decrease and death. In the original religion, mankind was required to separate the two realms carefully, and numerous taboos maintained this. The major smoke descending ritual was the funeral, which served to transport the soul from this world to the next. When a man died he was referred to as a "sick man" and the corpse was taken to the southern bedroom (that is, on the smoke descending side) of the house. After certain rites he was called a "dead man" and put in the central chamber. To make sure that the soul went to *puja*, the afterworld, a complicated death ceremony had to be held, maybe several years after the death when the family had amassed enough wealth to carry out the entire ritual properly. This included a large gathering of friends and family together with the slaughter of many buffalo, the spirit of one being responsible for taking the dead person's spirit to the next world. It was most important that the ceremony was carried out properly to ensure that the ancestor maintained an interest in the descendant's future prosperity.

There was thought to be a soul substance, with some living things such as man, rice and buffalo having a lot and others, such as frogs and the kapok tree, having only a little. The soul energy was the basis of both physical and spiritual strength and could be reinforced by eating things strong in soul spirit – hence the importance of rice, buffalo milk and meat as good things to eat to strengthen the soul energy. There were all sorts of other spirits such as *bombas*, which had an existence independent of the body and could be seen by psychic people. There were also *baitong*, people who lived normal lives with their family but who every so often would go out at night, make themselves invisible and take the heart from a living person, who would then sicken and die unless the heart was recoverd by a wizard. Unfortunately I didn't come across anyone who knew about or had seen any of these supernatural beings.

Christianity came to the Toraja with the Dutch when the original missionaries tried to oust completely what they saw as heathen beliefs. This effort was very unsuccessful and there were few converts, as the Toraja were loath to give up their death ceremony in view of its importance to them. Later the missionaries separated the idea of religion and custom and said that when the Toraja took Christian beliefs they did not necessarily have to give up their customs. A council in the early twentieth century decided on what was custom and what was belief and decreed that most of the smoke rising (that is, fertility) rituals were beliefs and the smoke descending ones, in particular the death ceremony, were customs, provided that when they conducted a death ceremony the Toraja did not actually reinforce the original beliefs that underpinned it. Thus when a Toraja converted to Christianity he could continue with certain rituals, in particular the death ceremony. This laid the foundation for ritual practices to flourish while the beliefs in which they were embedded waned. There were no widespread conversions to Christianity, however, until the 1950s when this took place as a response to fears that they might have to convert to the Muslim faith.

I wondered if this was why there seemed to be so little knowledge about the beliefs underpinning what the midwives did around birth, and why there was so little ceremony. I was therefore very pleased to be able to interview Indo Bura, who professed to be an animist, as I thought she might be able to enlighten me about these older beliefs. Unfortunately, however, she seemed rather ill at ease and either couldn't or wouldn't tell me very much about what she believed. I think this might have been because animists are now very much in the minority (25 per cent of the Toraja at most) and she may have felt embarrassed and maybe under pressure as a nonconformist in a mainly Christian environment.

Unlike the other midwives, Indo Bura had learnt how to do the work from her husband – both massage and traditional herbal medicine: "My husband was a medicine man and I used to watch him, and he also taught me. He died about five years ago and so now I have taken his place. I feel I am destined to help pregnant women and the god teaches me; this is just my feeling – there is no dream or anything." She didn't feel that this was anything which had been passed through the family, or that she had an obligation to pass it on to her children. Although she came into midwifery in rather a different way from the others I had spoken to, her treatment seemed very much the same, relying mainly on massage: "I do a lot of massage, usually from about the fifth month, whenever the woman feels like having it." During birth Indo Bura helped with massage, encouraging the woman to make herself as comfortable as possible in whatever way best suited her: "The position in which she gives birth depends entirely on the woman. If she is comfortable lying down, then she lies down; if she is comfortable squatting, then she squats – it's entirely up to her." Only if the birth was delayed would Indo Bura invoke spiritual help, promising that if everything went well the family would have a celebration, usually a meal and prayers to thank the god. Like other midwives she cut the umbilical cord with bamboo and buried the placenta, believing that if she didn't the baby would have an unfortunate life. For any problems with the birth, such as excess bleeding or breech, she massaged, although she felt that both problems were caused by the baby being in the wrong place and would not occur if the woman had come for regular massage. The majority of births happened with no problems, but if there was something serious and the mother had been in labour for several days she would take her to the hospital.

Although she was willing to send her clients to the hospital, Indo Bura did not feel as confident as Nek Reke about actually going to help her clients there: "If a woman goes to the hospital to give birth and then wants me to do the massage, I won't go because the doctors there will scold. They have to wait until they come back and then I'll go and do the massage in the house." As well as helping pregnant women Indo Bura could also deal with a number of other health problems, especially fevers in children. She used herbal remedies taught to her b her husband and prayed to the god before giving them to the patient. Like all the others she accepted whatever her clients offered in payment.

Our last visit was to Nek Minggu, whom we finally found tending her rice fields a long way from her house. She was a woman of about sixty with a kindly, weatherbeaten face who told us that she had been doing this work for about twenty years and still delivered an average of four babies a month. The work was very much part of her family tradition: "My mother was a *dukun* and so was my grandmother, and I learnt everything I know from them. Only when they both died did I start start helping pregnant women on my own. Before I started I had a dream when my dead grandmother came to me carrying a stone which she put in some water and then drank it after saying some words." Since then she hadn't had any more dreams of a similar kind, but said that as it was her grandmother who had visited her in the dream she couldn't teach women outside the family about the work. Unfortunately Nek Minggu's only daughter was not at all interested: "My daughter married a church person and she won't have anything to do with the prayers I use, so everything will die with me."

Massage was her main treatment, and she said that most women first came to her when they were about four months pregnant and visited her again maybe two or three times during the pregnancy. Most of the women were healthy and didn't have any problems, although she said some did bleed before the baby was due: "For this I give some very gentle massage and the bleeding usually stops. Maybe the baby gets into a better position." Unusually, for morning sickness she gave some water over which she had chanted some special prayers, which she said usually helped the woman feel a little better.

What she did to help women giving birth was very much like everyone else I had talked to and usually, she said, there were few problems. She had never seen a breech birth and put this down to the massage she did to get the baby into the right position. She said that sometimes she could tell whether it was going to be a boy or a girl as the stomach felt hard if it was going to be a boy and soft if it was going to be a girl, although as she quickly pointed out, this was not infallible! She said that most mothers didn't mind whether they had boys or girls, probably because descent can be traced bilaterally through both father and mother. Each person traces their ancestors on both the mother's and father's side, often identifying with the one to which he or she feels most attached. Sons and daughters have equal share of the inheritance, although to some degree this depends on their respective donations to the death feast.

Marriage used to be a very free and easy affair, although I didn't find out how Christianity had affected this. It was very casual, with couples living together and sealing the bond with a special sacrifice and feast only after they had been together for some time and had children. Those of higher rank might have an arranged marriage and be expected to keep together, but those of lower rank chose their own partners and divorce was very easy. While the Torajans were very severe about incest, killing those who indulged in it, illegitimacy was accepted very readily, the child living with its mother and becoming part of her family.

Nek Minggu had been called by some of her clients to the hospital to give them massage there, and she said that more women went to hospital to give birth nowadays: "Sometimes the hospital midwife will call to give me equipment, scissors and stuff like that. But I don't want it; I prefer to do things my way." People used to pay her with rice, but she said that nowadays most people give her money – the poor about 3,000 or 5,000 rupiah and the rich maybe 10,000. But like all the others, she would accept from her clients anything they were willing to give her.

PART III

LIVING IN
MALAYSIA

10

WHEN THE MIDWIFE IS A MAN: BIRTH AMONGST THE ORANG ASLI

DURING MY TRAVELS both within and outside Malaysia I had heard of male midwives, but De Ode was the first one I ever met. He was most amused that I should think this was anything unusual, for as he explained, it was the personality of the individual, not their sex, which determined whether they would be chosen by the spirits for this sort of work: "It is not unusual, amongst us Orang Asli, for a man to be a midwife. This is because we use spirits to help us in the birth, and spirits cannot be simply called to assist by just anyone. The spirit itself will choose whom it wants to communicate with and may decide on anyone it pleases. A person must be strong to communicate with a spirit, and the spirit knows whom it can depend on and will choose accordingly. Once the person is selected the spirit will communicate only with that person, and it will pass on all its knowledge to that person. When that person calls, the spirit will come to help." In the village of Mampas, De Ode was that person.

The name "Orang Asli" means literally "the original people" and is the name given to those who inhabit the far reaches of the tropical rainforest in Malaysia. There are now around 60,000 of them (in a total population of about 17 million), nearly two-thirds of whom still live in the more inaccessible jungle. Most of the rest live in rural but more accessible areas, and only a very few are part of the middle class with a professional job in an urban area. Getting to see them, especially in the more remote areas, is not easy, as many live in "restricted areas", areas of the jungle which are "off limits" to the general population because of so-called communist activity. At the same time the Government Department of Orang Asli Affairs (Jabatan Orang Asli, or JOA) is very protective of this group and is responsible both for their development and for ensuring that they are not exploited. I wanted very much to visit some Orang Asli in the more remote areas and began by approaching the JOA, only to be met with a wall of difficulties. I would be allowed to go only if I was part of a group of at least ten people with "a good reason for wanting to visit", and I would need to obtain a police permit before the JOA would even consider my request. Since the police permit was issued only for a specific visit at a certain time and date, and the JOA wouldn't say whether or not I could go until I had obtained the police permit, this was a catch-22 situation which I thought would probably take months to resolve. In the end it seemed easier just to confine myself to those Orang Asli who lived in more accessible areas which one didn't need special permission to visit.

In the above paragraphs I have spoken about the Orang Asli as if they are a homogeneous group, but in fact this is not so. Anthropologists usually divide the Orang Asli into three groups along physical and linguistic lines into Negritos, Senoi and Proto Malays. Even these groups, however, have within them some diversity of language, lifestyle and beliefs, and I found many local variations in the groups I visited, stemming partly from their original lifestyle and partly from the outside influences to which they had been exposed.

Kampong Durian, where I met De Ode, was not so inaccessible, although it was some miles down a narrow road which wound through rice *padi*, Malay kampongs and a rubber plantation, eventually coming to an abrupt end at the village. Arifin, who had introduced me to the first midwife, Buleh, came with us to introduce us to the *batin* or headman of the village. He was a dissolute-looking man with very red eyes, who even at 10 a.m. was smelling strongly of alcohol. At first he was not at all keen to talk, and I began to wonder whether we were going to get anywhere here – the Orang Asli are known to be very shy and often won't talk to strangers. Finally De Ode (who, we found out later, was the *batin*'s brother) turned up, and he was as charming and outgoing as the *batin* was surly and introverted. He invited us over to his house, which stood on the edge of the village surrounded by flowering bushes and fruit trees. Underneath it lived various families of cats and dogs.

Sitting in the cool of his wooden house, he told me how he came to know the spirits who were of such importance for his work as a healer: "The spirit teaches through dreams, and that is how I first came to know of them. We call the spirit Raib and it is like the wind, it cannot be seen, but we know that it is good and will help us when we need it. The delivery of a child is easy when this spirit is around." To contact a spirit, prayers have to be performed and these are often in the form of songs, which have long stories, each spirit having a different song which will be sung when its help is needed. For the spirits which help during a birth, however, a different technique is required: "To call the spirit for those mothers who are going to give birth the song is not sung but whispered, as you mustn't make any noise." To demonstrate this, De Ode then sang me a song which he sings to contact the spirit which helps people who are critically ill: "In this song I am asking the spirit to help clear whatever illness there is in the body and to make the sick person well again. This singing is like praying, and after it the spirit will come in like the wind and help cure the illness. This song was taught to me by my father." He sang to the accompaniment of a simple guitar made of bamboo, about two feet in length and six inches in circumference, which had a considerable sentimental and spiritual value for him: "This guitar is mine; I made it, and I think I am the only one in my tribe who has such an instrument. I will never part with it; not for any price." The instrument had a nasal, haunting sound, and even after all this time I have only to close my eyes for it to re-echo through my mind again.

151

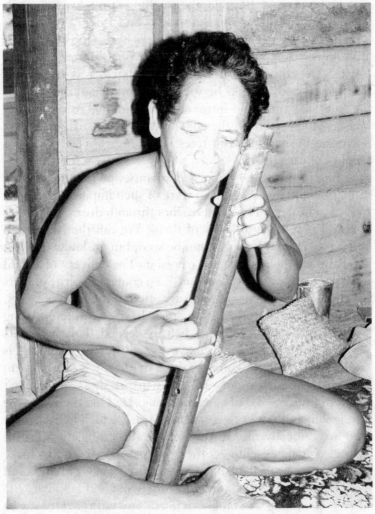

De Ode singing to the spirits

While De Ode was concerned with the spirits it was his stepmother, Tihol, who provided the practical help, both being necessary for a successful birth. Tihol was very shy and talked to me with a group of women who helped her answer the questions and gave her moral support; these included De Ode's wife, child and grandchildren. She told me how she had learnt her craft: "I learnt the art of midwifery from my father, who died when I was about twenty years old. Having seen my father attend to women, I naturally picked up how to do it. We think of it as a community service rather than something for which we get paid." She felt that you had to be a special sort of person to be a midwife: "To be a midwife you have to be brave and you have to be courageous because of the child and having to make quick decisions. I do not use the help of a spirit myself and I don't say any of the prayers. If that is necessary I get De Ode."

For most women birth was easy and quick; some of the women had been in labour for as long as two days, but everyone agreed that this was extremely unusual. Most thought that a labour of an hour or so was about normal, and as in so many of the other groups they seemed to be defining this in terms of the second stage only. I was surprised how many of them seemed to discount the first stage completely! Herbs were given before and after birth: "There are four types of root which are given to the mother during confinement and which we continue to give her for seven days after birth. This strengthens the body and lessens the flow of blood." De Ode was obviously the village expert on this and said that people came to him from far and wide for his herbal remedies: "There are many different types of *akar kayu*. Different types of roots are mixed together for different types of ailments. We have remedies for diabetes, high blood pressure, hardened arteries, and so on." After giving birth the mother would be massaged, although the massage did not have the importance it has for some groups. There were a few dietary restrictions: "After birth the mother is given ginger to eat, and two days after delivery she is given some chicken. The old practice was to feed her with monkey meat, which is good for the blood and tastes a bit like mutton, but now chicken is given instead as monkeys are hard to find." There was no exclusion period when the mother was restricted to the house, but she was not normally allowed to bathe until three days after the birth.

Tihol went on to explain how she dealt with the umbilical cord and placenta: "The umbilical cord is cut with a sharp

153

bamboo and I use turmeric to clean the area where the cut is made. I tie the cord with two pieces of string a few inches apart before the cut is made. In the old days we used to use plant fibres rather than string." The placenta was then buried near the house, either underneath it or to one side. Generally it was felt that there were not many problems, and that minor ones at least could be helped with their own herbal remedies. There was a special herb which could be used for excessive bleeding (meriat) and a retained placenta would be encouraged to separate and be expelled with massage.

Despite the confidence which they seemed to show in their remedies, they were careful to point out that they did use the government midwife: "Of course now, with modern methods, there is less dependence on the herbs. We now have the assistance of doctors and our midwife is used only when the doctor is not available. We still retain the old methods; if we are in difficulties and we cannot get a doctor, we use our midwife. We believe in passing on the traditions so that they are not forgotten." As Tihol had said previously, the help she gave was considered a social service rather than something for which she would expect payment. Nevertheless she did receive payment at the celebration of the baby's first birthday – the only birthday the Orang Asli celebrate: "A year after the baby is born, a special celebration is given where the midwife will receive gifts for helping in the delivery. She normally gets $7, a mirror and clothes, plus a coconut which is tied four times with a red thread. I think the coconut is symbolic of the womb and the red string represents blood, but unfortunately we have forgotten the significance of this ceremony and many of the other traditional ways of the tribe."

I was surprised at the confidence these women displayed in their ability to control their own fertility. As they explained to me, abortion was unnecessary as they had herbs both to help them conceive and to prevent conception: "We don't carry out abortions here because we don't need to. We have special herbs which we use as contraception; they are special mushrooms and roots which must be taken every day for one month by the women. We also have medicine if anyone has difficulty in getting pregnant." The women were absolutely confident that these remedies worked, although when I asked them how many children they hoped to have, the answer was "the more the merrier". It seemed, therefore, that if these remedies were not 100 per cent effective, it wasn't something they would greatly worry about.

The people in this village were part of the Temuan group, which is itself part of the Proto Malay group. They tend to be more settled than some of the other Orang Asli groups, and this village had in fact been there since 1926. It had its own rubber plantation in which many of the villagers worked, and they also grew much of their own food. They lived close to the Malays but seemed to have retained their own culture to a very large degree. After we had talked to De Ode and Tihol we were invited on a fishing expedition to a nearby stream. Skidding down a deep bank, we watched as all the young people splashed around in the water feeling under the large boulders to make the fish swim into their small baskets. Unfortunately an hour's work provided only one very small and inedible fish, although it was agreed that a good time had been had by all. As we walked around the banks of the river De Ode showed me many different plants, seemingly pulling them at random from the undergrowth and telling me what their roots and leaves could be used for. He said that many of the herbs he used only grew deep in the jungle and that as so much of it had now disappeared, finding them was getting more and more difficult. To him the profuse vegetation was a storehouse of cures for every conceivable type of illness.

Arifin told us that eight kilometres further into the jungle there was another village of Temuans that he knew and a few weeks later, having managed to acquire a four-wheel-drive vehicle, we drove along the rutted track to the village of Langkap. We were lucky that it hadn't rained in the previous few days, as the track would have been impassable in any sort of vehicle. Slowly we negotiated the longitudinal ruts, once having to lurch over rather sickeningly to go round a tree growing at a 45-degree angle out of the nearby bank. Stopping to recover from these experiences, we were surprised to see a car coming towards us in the opposite direction. It was surprising not only to see a car so deep in the jungle, but one that was going at a speed which suggested a motorway rather than the track we had just negotiated so slowly and with so much effort. We began to wonder if the bad quality of the track was all in our minds!

The vilage was spread over a large area, with houses having been built wherever there was a suitable clearing rather than to conform to any kind of collective pattern. The twentieth century had arrived here in the form of mains electricity and sacks of concrete and corrugated iron waiting, presumably, to be turned into buildings. Many of the houses, however, were built entirely in the traditional way on stilts with *attap* walls and roofs. This mixture of the traditional and the modern was found not only in the physical surroundings but also in the thoughts and ideas of the villagers – this was evident once I started talking to them.

Nau was a young man in his late twenties and I spoke to him and his seventy-year-old father Garadas, who had a tremendous fund of stories about what it was like in the jungle during the Japanese occupation in World War II. Unfortunately, the person in this village who knew the most about birth had gone away for a while but as Nau said, everyone here knew how to cope with an ordinary birth: "In this village we don't have a particular person who is the midwife. Anyone who knows and understands childbirth will help." In most cases this meant some older person in the family: "There are usually old people around who have the experience and know what to do, and they will come and help if there is a need. The *batin*, who is my wife's grandfather, helps with deliveries, and it was my wife's father who came and helped when my wife gave birth to our last child a few months ago."

The whole process of birth seemed very much the same as in Kampong Mampas, although here they seemed to have taken over some of the ideas and practices of the nearby Malay kampongs. One of these was the *pantang*, an exclusion period of forty-four days during which the woman avoids certain foods and doesn't leave the house. The foods avoided, however, were not the same as those rejected by the Malays and reflected the different diets of the two communities: "During our *pantang* of forty-four days the mother doesn't eat *musang* [civet cat], *knachil* [mousedeer], wild goat, ripe bananas, beef, *chilli api* [literally chilli fire, the very small, very hot chillies] and certain types of fish. The reason we forbid all these foods is that they could cause her to bleed and thus endanger her life." Whoever had helped with the birth also undertook a ritual washing, another practice found amongst some Malays: "Once the baby has been born we give some special water to the *bidan* to wash his hands. We pound some rice, lime, coconut leaves and dengin leaves; we mix this with water and give it to the midwife to wash his hands. This is to throw away any bad luck and also like cleansing himself because of all that blood and everything is dirty."

Unusually for an Orang Asli community, the people in this village traced their descent through the mother, probably having copied this from the surrounding small groups of Minangkabau Malays. As Nau explained, "We prefer daughters because we follow the *adat perpatih*, where the property is passed down to the daughters rather than the sons. When the son gets married he goes to his wife's house to stay." Nau was also very amusing in discussing whether it was possible to tell before birth whether the baby was going to be a boy or a girl. He began by saying quite confidently that an experienced midwife could tell whether a baby was a boy or a girl by the way they were lying: "A female always lies straight and the male slanting." After thinking about it for a minute or two he said that they are not invariably right – sometimes they do get it wrong!

Nau then went on to tell me in some detail about the urinary infection that all the men were very scared of getting from their wives after they had given birth. Some thought that this disease could be caught just by stepping on a place where a woman had recently urinated. Fortunately there is a cure which Nau described as "number one *akar kayu*", which he was able to go and get for me as he had the plants growing just outside his house. This was also given to women just after they had given birth: "It consists of the roots of the kelimau, kebangunun and the bark of the durian tree, which are all boiled together. We strain the water and give it to the woman just after she has given birth, but only after the placenta and everything has come out. This will prevent her getting the woman's disease as well as heavy periods. If she doesn't take it she may pass on her sickness to the man. The men take this *akar kayu* when they get the men's disease – pain in the stomach and difficulty and pain with urinating."

Nau answered all my questions as fully as he could, with great earnestness. I never cease to be amazed and sometimes very touched at just how helpful many of my respondents are in trying to answer and make sense of questions which must seem very odd to them. This is particularly true in traditional societies, where there is a lot of "taken-for-granted" knowledge and actions, and where different ways of doing things are not necessarily discussed and evaluated – especially, it seems, concerning events like giving birth. I often tried too hard to give meanings to everything and to assign a significance to actions when there was none. Nau, for instance, went on to explain that the placenta would be buried near the house, this being done in the morning if the baby was born at night. He was amused at the idea that there might be some significance about this timing: "Oh no! There is no significance to this; it's just that at night it's too dark to see what we are doing, so we wait until the morning, when it is brighter." Well! I just felt that I had to ask!

In this village people seemed to be much less concerned with the spirits, and Nau felt that this was a result of government interference. The aid provided by the JOA, he thought, was making the people lazy and encouraging them to forget their traditional ways. He was very concerned, and was attempting to remedy the situation by trying to learn the prayers and songs from the old people who still remembered them, but was very frustrated by his inability to learn: "My grandfather and father-in-law tried to teach me the *jampi*, but it simply doesn't seem to go into my head. You have to remember the words by heart and you cannot miss out a single word when you are doing the *jampi*. You cannot become a *bomoh* [medicine man] by just learning two or three kinds of *jampi*; there are so many. That is one reason why the *jampi* method is not used so much now; nowadays the youngsters turn towards modern medicine." He couldn't understand why this should be so, but maybe he, too, had come under the modern influences which made it difficult to tune into the traditional ways of doing things.

Like the villagers in Kampong Durian, the women were confident that they could control their fertility, although as Nau said, women rarely resorted to traditional remedies, which were now very difficult to find: "We have *akar kayu* which can prevent pregnancy for two or three years, or there is some which can prevent you from getting pregnant for ever, but the herbs are very difficult to get so now most people take the family planning tablets which are provided by the government." As a result the number of births in the village had fallen considerably and often no babies were born for two or three years. I wondered if it had also changed the way decisions about whether or not to have children were made. Nau's wife had just recently given birth to a child: "I have two children; the eldest is four and the youngest two months old. I asked my wife whether she wanted another child and she said yes, so we did. We both have to agree before having a new baby, and if she didn't want to we wouldn't. If we can afford it we'd like five children altogether. But of course we don't want to have them all too quickly."

Women could, of course, go to the hospital for birth, but this had serious financial implications for anyone who decided to do so: "Only those who can afford it go to the hospital to give birth because the JOA usually send us to the hospital in Kuala Lumpur [about 60 kilometres away] by helicopter. This is free, but after that if we want to visit our wife we have to use our own money to travel. So that's why most of us prefer to give birth here." Because of this the

159

village women much preferred to give birth at home and would use the hospital only in an emergency. Nau was not convinced that this sort of service made them any healthier, and seemed very divided as to whether progress of this kind was real progress if the traditional ways of the villagers were being left behind: "Compared to before I would say there are more deaths now. Last year there were three deaths of babies three to four months old, but in those days we very seldom had deaths like this. This is because in those days we always did *jampi* for the sickness but now everyone takes hospital medicine and the *jampi* is reduced." I felt that Nau was poised between the traditional and the modern, neither of one nor the other and not sure that he belonged with either.

In my quest to find more remote Orang Asli villages I went to Tula, which could be approached only by boat, as it was on an island in the middle of a complex of lakes and swamps on the east coast of the Malaysian peninsula. There was a rickety platform which had been built over a marsh on to which we had to climb and then walk (or in my case wobble rather nervously) on slippery logs that had been put end to end over the rest of the swamp. I was sure the locals, and especially the children, would be able to run along these logs quite easily, and I was glad there was no one obviously watching my halting progress!

We came eventually to a small clearing where there were four houses, all built on stilts and one built entirely of *attap* rather than wooden planks. It was extremely quiet and at first we thought no one was there until a man came on to the veranda and looked at us with quizzical amusement. He didn't seem in the least perturbed by our little party and sat down to answer Letchimi's questions as if this were the sort of thing he did every day. Tau was a man of about forty-five and in his lifetime he had experienced many changes in his way of living: "When I was a child we used to be so frightened of outsiders visiting us. The minute we saw a boat coming towards our place we would all run into the jungle to hide.

Sometimes I would stay sitting in my hut, but then I too would run off when they got nearer. At that time we always thought they were coming to kill us." This belief was not fanciful, as it was not unknown for the Orang Asli to be taken as slaves by the Malays, and the impact of both the Japanese during World War II and the Communists during the communist insurgency made them even more distrustful of strangers. He talked, somewhat regretfully, of the kind of life he had lived as a child in the jungle, which was no longer possible in the reduced area of the forest now available: "In those days we used to be able to live in the jungle however we wanted. I can remember that we used to be able to live on this special sort of potato. It was long and big and all we needed to do was slice a little piece of the potato off and roast it over the fire and eat it. One person could live on just one potato for three or four months. I can't seem to find that kind of potato in the jungle these days and I often wonder what's happened to them."

He went on to talk about birth in the times when much of his life was spent travelling in the rainforest: "Women followed their husbands deep into the jungle to look for food. If a woman were pregnant she would give birth there by herself, although of course she would have her husband's help. They would stay in one spot for maybe a week, and after that they would continue walking with the baby. Wherever they were in the jungle the couple would just give birth; there would be no midwife or anyone else around to help." With a more settled existence, this was something else which had changed: "Nowadays whenever anyone wants to give birth she'll go across to the village [just across the lake], which is where the midwife lives. But most men and women here do know what to do."

Tau's grandfather had been the village *bomoh*, and he had many stories to relate of the cures that he had seen this old man bring about. Even today people came from the nearby towns to his grandfather for cures to illnesses which ordinary doctors had not been able to cope with. Tau himself had a wide knowledge of the jungle and the various ways in which it could be used to provide food, shelter and medicines, but he discounted this knowledge in the light of what his children had achieved with a more conventional education: "I didn't go to school, but nowadays most of our children do so. I have three children; they went to school and now two of them are married. The younger generation are all clever because they all go to school; they also mix with outsiders and learn a lot, but we, the older generation, we have our experiences and that is all." He had moved to this more inaccessible place because it was more peaceful, and although it was surrounded by rubber trees rather than the jungle, he felt that it provided him with what he poetically described as the necessities of a happy life: "Where there is a mountain, where there is jungle, where there is a blowpipe; that is my place."

At Tau's suggestion we went across the lake to the village, where he said we would find the midwife used by many of the women in the area. Chino was in her eighties and had difficulty with her eyes, and although she was a little shy at first she was very pleased to talk to us sitting under the shade of the mango tree just by the house where she lived with her son and daughter. Like Tau, she had seen many changes: "I was born and brought up here, but of course in those days it was very different. There was a lot more jungle around before the authorities moved in." There were medical facilities provided by the government, but according to her most of the women in the village continued to help each other out during birth, much as they had always done: "Most of the women here know the midwife's work because they are always present when a child is born and they watch what she does. This is how I learnt, by watching my mother do it. When I was young I used to do it on my own, but now with my failing sight I just help others do it, especially if there are problems."

Problems were not, however, expected and rarely encountered and birth, like other "rites of passage", was a simple affair. There were no ceremonies for birth (or marriage), although since the Orang Asli lived a more settled existence closer to the Malays, some of Malay ideas had been introduced. The *pantang*, for instance, was something new: "In those days there were no prohibitions; after giving birth a woman would eat anything she could get in the jungle." Similarly the free and easy attitudes towards marriage had also changed – as Tau had put it: "If a boy sleeps with a girl and she doesn't mind, then they are considered married." Chino confirmed this, but added: "Nowadays some of the youngsters like to follow the Malay style and have a *bersanding* – a fairly elaborate ceremony where the married couple become "king and queen for a day" and are dressed very sumptuously, and all the members of the family come to bless them.

I always felt a considerable empathy with the Orang Asli groups I visited. I liked the equable nature of their groups and the way in which they seemed to live so much in harmony both with the environment and with each other. Although they were often rather shy at first, once we started talking their warmth would become apparent. The group that affected me the most, however, were the nomadic Batek group which I was lucky enough to see and talk with in Taman Negara, a park of protected tropical rainforest in central Malaysia. Much of the forest where the Batek live has disappeared, but there are still around 2,000 of them who hunt, fish and gather food in the jungle as they have always done.

When we went to the park the only way to get there was by boat on one of the huge rivers that meander through the forest. It provided a wonderful introduction to the park as the cultivated rubber and oil palm gradually gave way to the profusion of huge jungle trees which are so characteristic of untouched rainforest in this part of the world. At that time a new road was being built which, it was said, would cut down the time it takes to get to the park and encourage more people to visit. I couldn't help thinking what a pity it would be when the road was open and people would be able to roar up in their cars, presumably destroying the peace with their noise and fumes. The immensity of the rainforest is somehow easier to appreciate from a boat rather than a car, and I fear that the environmental groups are correct when they say that the road will destroy something of this last Malaysian wilderness. After three hours or so (which included half an hour to mend a breakdown on the boat) we arrived at the park centre and climbed up a huge flight of steps to the jetty. It was difficult to imagine that in the rainy season the river rose right to the top of these steps. At the top was the administration centre for the park, with a camping site and chalets from which it was possible to explore the forest on foot and by boat.

One of the nice things about Taman Negara is that you can walk along jungle paths and therefore experience the jungle without the hassle and hard work of having to hack your way through the undergrowth and without getting lost. I am told that if the jungle has never been logged there is very little undergrowth, but nowadays it is very difficult to find unlogged jungle except in this park. Walking along the paths I had a wonderful sense of the jungle's denseness; of all the different things growing in a primitive effusion of life energy. I don't see it as a struggle one against the other, but rather as a cacophony of different things which can't help but bump into each other and affect each other because of their close proximity. The jungle feels very closed in and even after a little while it is difficult to tell where you are, how far away things are, and it wasn't long before I had completely lost my sense of direction.

We had been told that a group of Orang Asli were staying quite close to the centre, and although we met one or two of them while we were out walking we could never engage them in conversation. They would walk past with a certain bouncy purposefulness and ignore us completely; it was as if we didn't exist, and perhaps for them we didn't. I thought we might have more luck if we could engage an Orang Asli guide who might know them and with whom they might feel sufficiently at ease to talk to us. For various reasons this wasn't possible, and instead we were introduced to Mohammed who, although not an Orang Asli, had lived all his life in the park and knew them very well. He came to see us sporting a rather punky hairstyle and designer trousers – not how I would expect a guide to look! He seemed very cheerful and friendly and said that we were in luck because a group of Bateks had been in the vicinity of the centre for the last week or two. Apparently this happened only infrequently as most of the time they were much further away and more difficult to contact.

He turned up on the day of our trek in a very fetching pair of what looked like designer shorts and an even more fetching Tyrolean hat made of leather. This was an original, a souvenir from Germany, where he had been sent on a language course. He was obviously quite amused by my trekking clothes, which consisted of jungle boots with socks turned over the top and a dress. It was the best way of dressing that I could think of which would keep me reasonably cool yet protect my feet and ankles from the leeches. As we waited on the jetty for the boat that was going to take us up one of the rivers, Mohammed told us how he had spent all his life in the park, his father having been one of the first forest rangers appointed after the park had been set up by the British. He had spent a lot of his childhood going out into the forest with his father, which was how he had learnt so much about it. Until the last five years few people had come to the park and even fewer had made the four-day jungle trek to the top of Gunan Tahan, the highest mountain in Malaysia, which is in the middle of Taman Negara. Although more people now came to visit it could be a lonely place in which to live, especially during the rainy season when it would be cut off from everyone, as even the boats sometimes could not negotiate the swollen rivers.

Going up the river by boat was wonderful; huge trees leant out across the water, their enormous bulk counterweighted by the root systems which spread out and embraced the bank. Despite their size and seeming impregnability they can be prooted quite easily. In the rainy season, when the water rises 10 feet or more, trees come down and sometimes cause a landslide, and as we went along the river we saw many remains of dead trees. Where the water was shallow it had

165

a lovely coppery glow and we could easily see the stones at the bottom. Where it was deeper it had an inky, oily look, especially where there were no rapids, but the seeming stillness of the water belied the strong current.

We didn't have to go very far before we came to where the Orang Asli group were staying, its presence indicated by one of the women washing in the river. She was small with short curly hair shaved off over the forehead, on which she had put flowers. She grinned at Mohammed as we climbed up a steep bank and came upon a group of their houses in a small clearing. I suppose the best way of describing these houses would be as "lean-tos". They consisted of several large pieces of bamboo which had been lashed together to make a tent shape, on to which various leaves and branches were woven. The houses were enclosed only on one side, although there was a deep eave at the front to keep off the rain. Most of them had just a woven mat on the floor, although one of them had a very small platform. I was very excited to see that one of the women had what looked like a very new baby. I asked how old he was, but she couldn't remember exactly when he was born, and after discussing it with everyone else in the group decided he was probably about thirteen days old.

Everyone obviously knew and accepted Mohammed and, as I had hoped, were willing to accept and talk to us. If we had just turned up and started trying to talk to them on our own, I don't think we would have stood a chance.

Sitting there in front of this simple house, with people who had so little in the way of material possessions, I was acutely aware of the difficulties of my approach. How could I ever do more than slightly indent the fabric of their lives? There were three or four families in this group who lived and did everything together. I was struck by the feeling of their interconnectedness not only with the forest but also with each other. They seemed to be totally absorbed with each other as they went about their daily tasks. One man was carefully making a blowpipe, heating it up in the fire which burnt outside his house and checking it every few minutes to see that it was straight. The others sat around smoking

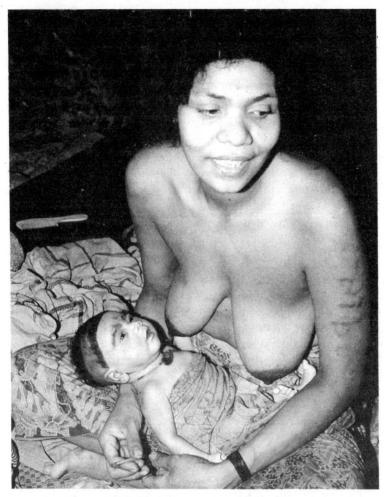

Tijah with her newborn baby

and laughing with each other and giving us sideways looks every now and then. Their possessions were very few indeed, although one person [the one making the blowpipe] did have a radio. But mostly it was just one pot for cooking and a few odds and ends which were kept at the back of their houses.

For them pregnancy was nothing special but just an ordinary part of life – as Tijah, who had just given birth, explained: "We don't eat anything special or do anything

167

different when we are pregnant. We don't have any special ceremonies for the mother or the baby. When we give birth we go to another place not far from here [in fact she showed us later, and it was just across the river], where we build a special small hut. Only the womenfolk will be around. The husband will be outside and he will come in only if it looks as if it could be serious and the mother might not survive. But so far that situation has never arisen with us. It takes about twenty or thirty minutes to give birth, and once everything is over we come back to our houses here. If the mother gets stomach pains before birth we apply the meriam leaf [which we get from the jungle]. We just slightly burn the leaf and then pad it around her stomach while it is still hot."

They were obviously rather amused at my questions and roared with laughter when I asked them in what position they gave birth. I thought this might have been embarrassment but I felt much more that it was not, according to them, something which one would normally find it necessary to discuss. One gave birth in whatever position was dictated by the energy of the moment. They dealt with the umbilical cord and placenta in the traditional way: "We cut the umbilical cord with bamboo and we then bury it with the placenta. Part of the umbilical cord we tie on to a piece of string, which we then tie round the baby's hand. We also shave off a little of the baby's hair and wrap it is a small piece of cloth, which we tie around the baby's neck. We do this to protect it from the spirits which cause illness." She showed me how the newborn baby had been given this treatment.

"After the mother has given birth we give her three kinds of root medicine. We don't know the name of them but again we get them from the jungle." Her husband pointed to where the herbs had been pushed into the thatching of their roof: "We also do the massage for the mother for two or three days to help her feel good. After birth, for two or three weeks the mother doesn't eat salty, oily or sour food; not even sour fruit." After giving birth, they said, there were rarely any problems: "Sometimes the milk doesn't flow properly and then we pad the breasts with meriam leaves and massage them." For more difficult problems and illness, generally a more experienced person would be called in the shape of the local *bomoh*: "When there is any illness among us we call the *bomoh* to cure it. He'll make the sick person sit in the middle and everyone else around. Then he'll sing the song which calls the spirit to take away the illness. The *bomoh* is somewhere in the jungle and we go and look for him when we want him. But usually the illness is not very serious, so we do everything ourselves." The *bomoh* is an extremely important person in this group, as he is the link between the earth and the spirits which control both individual and group well-being. Although one of the women said that she was "the midwife", I think this was probably just to please me, for as she said, "All the women in this group know what to do. I learnt what to do from my mother, but most women can do it because we are always there together when a child is being born."

I realized how difficult it would be to befriend and really get to know a group such as this. They are an intensely private people who seem to be an organic whole, with many things not needing to be said. One would need to experience this within their context of the forest if one were really to get to know them. As we sat and talked to them the modern world, in the shape of husky young people carrying huge rucksacks, walked along the path not 50 feet from their houses. These outsiders seemed to cause not a ripple within the dense network of these Batek lives, and I'm not sure whether they even saw them. It was as if they were so totally absorbed in the bubble of their own lives that there was no time or space for such alien influences,

They were obviously quite surprised and often amused by my questions, many of which I felt they couldn't see the point of. To say they live unconsciously is to give the misleading impression that they are somehow underdeveloped and thoughtless. They did not, however, question and justify what they did, as we might; instead they seemed to have a deep sense of rightness, which for them was justification enough. The idea of discussing various actions which could be taken in different situations and evaluating which would be best seemed entirely foreign to their life. In general life went on much as always, with very little concession to modernity. It had, however, touched them in terms of the lucrative opportunities now available for guiding tourists up the mountain, although Mohammed told us that they would do this only if they felt like it. The effects on the group as a whole, however, seemed very modest, as Tijah said: "Our food is mainly plain rice or some kind of yam which we find in the river. We also hunt animals like squirrels and monkeys with our blowpipes. Sometimes we also guide the tourists to Gunung Tahan and when that person gets paid he will buy food for the whole group – he might go to the shop and buy sardines or something like that,"

11

A TRADITION UNDER THREAT: TRADITIONAL MIDWIFERY IN THE MALAY KAMPONGS

READ ANY TOURIST brochure about Malaysia, and the virtues of life on the east coast of the peninsula are sure to be extolled. Here, one can experience the Western idea of a lotus-eating tropical paradise: relax in the serenity and calm of the Malay villages or kampongs, spend all day basking on the glorious sandy but empty beaches, and forget about the cares of the other world that you have left. This tourist idyll, however, is only one aspect of this part of Malaysia. For the Malays the east coast is seen as the cradle, the nurturer and the preserver of Malay culture. Here it was, in the small kampongs dotted along the coast and along the river banks, that the traditional Malay life was lived: where rice and the other simple necessities of life were grown; where birth, life and death followed a prescribed pattern; where everyone knew their place and life followed its relatively predictable course. Malaysia is one of the more industrialized countries of the region, but life in these east coast kampongs seems to continue much as it has always done.

For many a Malay working in government offices in Kuala Lumpur, on the more developed west coast, the east coast kampong epitomizes both the world he or she has lost and the place from which his or her roots are derived. There is often a strong sentimantal connection with the original home in the kampong, and on any festival – especially an important one like Hari Raya Puasa, after the Ramadan fast – the streets of Kuala Lumpur will be empty of Malays, who will all have returned to their kampongs. For many, therefore, the east coast is a symbol of Malay identity in terms of culture, lifestyle and politics.

There is, however, another, darker side to all these positive aspects, for it is here that most of the poverty in West Malaysia is to be found. For the farmers it is a struggle to grow enough to feed their families, and many are very poor. Unlike the more equable west coast, the east coast has a monsoon season during which many kampongs are flooded, necessitating that whole villages move elsewhere for a while. Where the floods will be most severe cannot be predicted, and most years there is some loss of life in the worst-hit areas. During the monsoon most farming and fishing activities cease, adding to the financial strains of the subsistence farmer. Even if there are no floods it can rain for three or more days on end with a soaking tropical downpour which makes just the tasks of ordinary living difficult and uncomfortable. This is the other, darker, side to the tropical idyll put forward in the travel brochures.

Malay midwives, or *bidans*, have a very good reputation amongst all the different ethnic groups who live in Malaysia. To meet some I went to stay in Kampong Pemuda, a coastal kampong situated on the very edge of the sea on a peninsula of sand jutting out from the mainland. There was the beach, as empty and gloriously sandy as the brochures had promised, behind which stretched a belt of coconut palms. The kampong consisted of traditional Malay houses strung out on either side of the road which wound up the middle of the peninsula through the village. All the houses were built in the traditional Malay pattern: of wooden planks on stilts with a kitchen area on the ground at the back. It looked as if each person had chosen his or her place to build a house; some houses had been extended in various directions to add new rooms. There were no gardens, although most houses had trees or bushes growing around them depending on how close they were to the sea and how sandy the soil was. Scrubby grass grew everywhere, and goats and chickens roamed around between and under the houses; as the people were Muslims, no one owned either pigs or dogs. As we slowly drove through the village, children looked at us with undisguised interest while their parents, often from the shade of their verandas, eyed us more circumspectly.

The house where we stayed was right at the end of the village, a hundred yards or more from the last house in a long row. From the outside it looked like the other houses and had once, we were later to learn, been owned by the Chinese towkay who owned the boats and the fish-processing unit in which all the villagers used to work. The family had since gone on to better things (although one member ran a shop a few miles from the village) and the house had been leased to the Malayan Nature Society, who were doing it up so that people like us could stay in it. The main part was still in very good order and certain mod cons – like a pump to bring water from the well to a tank, and a proper bathroom – had recently been installed. As throughout the village, electricity was available only from dusk to about midnight, but that was easy to live with.

And so we settled down to kampong living. Much to Emma's delight, the goats soon realized that food was to be had from us and came round in the mornings bleating for any scraps on offer. Housekeeping was remarkably easy, as any sand brought into the house could simply be swept away through the cracks in the floorboards to the ground underneath. At first insects were a pest; I had my arms covered in ants when I took out of the cupboard two plates between which someone had left some sugar. When we first arrived the mosquitoes and sandflies were extremely voracious, although Letchimi thought that the house was relatively insect-free! I've never discovered why Western foreigners seem to make such heavy weather of the insects compared with the locals. Is it that we have thinner skin or more desirable blood? Or do the locals just notice them less? With judicious use of mosquito coils and regular sweeping they became much less annoying as the week wore on, or perhaps we just didn't bother about them so much.

It was not long before we discovered that one of the kampong midwives lived just a few houses away from where we were staying. Wan Limah was a very cheerful and voluble woman who I thought at first was much younger than her fifty-three years. She lived in a typical Malay house; I climbed up the steps to a large room (usually called the hall, although it is invariably the sitting area) along both sides of which were entrances to different rooms used by some of her five daughters and their husbands. Like so many of the Malay *bidans*, she had learnt from a female relative: "In the beginning I used to help my cousin, who was a *bidan*. Wherever she went I followed and helped her, and that's how I learnt." At first she said that women didn't come to see her until they were in labour and ready to give birth, but it was clear that although this happened with some women, many others came to her whenever they felt the need: "Sometimes women do come to me in early pregnancy to find out how many months pregnant they are, and I can tell them just by touching and feeling the stomach. I know each month how the baby will be if I feel the stomach." Later in the pregnancy women would come to her to check that the baby was in the correct position in which to be born, and making sure about this was one of the most important things the *bidan* would do. It might have been one of the reasons why Limah rarely had to deal with a breech birth: "They come to me when they are eight or nine months pregnant to check the position of the child. If it is in the wrong position then I will *jampi* some coconut oil and rub the stomach slowly and gently turn the baby back to the right position. I will also say some holy words while doing this."

While many women may not come to Limah until they are in labour, this does not mean that they are completely isolated or unsupported during the pregnancy. Even in the unlikely event that some members of the family will not be living either in the same house or nearby, they will be well steeped in the

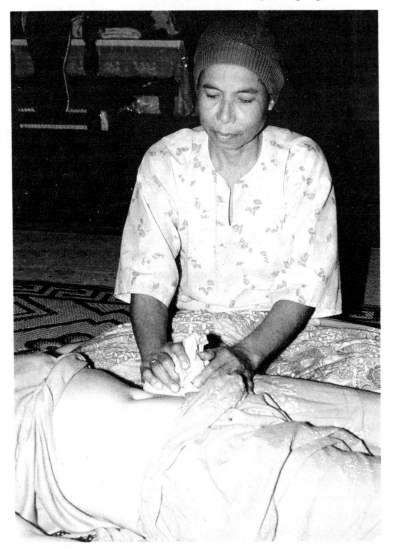

Wan Limah using a tuku ball to massage the author's stomach

local system of traditional health. This provides them with all the information they need to keep healthy during pregnancy and birth; especially afterwards, when both mother and baby are thought to be at special risk. In this traditional system a healthy body is thought to be one which is neither too hot nor cold and is therefore in physical, psychological and spiritual harmony. Illness occurs when for various reasons the body may become overheated or too cold, and the cure will then be to eat hot or cold foods to restore its equilibrium. When I first came to Malaysia I was very confused when people talked about hot and cold foods, as I thought at first that this referred to the temperature at which the food was eaten, when in fact it refers to the food's intrinsic qualities. An experienced Malay *bomoh* can, by taking pulse readings, looking at the patient and finding out about the symptoms, say very precisely in what way the body is hot or cold and what needs to be done to restore its equilibrium. The causes of such imbalances may be both supernatural and physical, so that for a cure to be obtained various rituals may be required as well as changes in diet.

For the average Malay, this traditional system provides a framework in which it is possible to cure simple diseases and to deal with events like pregnancy, birth and after. I have described this system as if it were fixed and unchanging, but this is not how it works in practice. Carol Laderman, an anthropologist who lived in an east coast kampong for fifteen months researching traditional midwifery and diet, found that the system had a considerable dynamism. Thus, apart from a few staple foods such as fish and rice, there was only very general agreement – and quite a lot of disagreement – about what constituted hot and cold foods. For example, hot foods consisted of fats, spices, animal protein, salty and bitter foods, while cold foods were generally considered to be juicy fruits and vegetables that needed a lot of water for growth, together with those that were slimy and tasted sour. The mainstays of the diet, rice and fish, were considered neutral, although some species of fish were classified according to whether they were hot or cold. There was yet another class of foods called *biasa* foods which were those which intensified already existing disharmonies. To a large degree this was a very individual thing which depended on the person's general level of health, age, and so on, and how the different foods reacted within that person.

Carol Laderman found that when she talked to people about this, individuals had no compunction whatsoever in reclassifying food if they felt that it was right for their particular situation. At different times of the day and at different seasons, foods could change their hot or cold effects. It was generally agreed, however, that whereas pregnancy was a period of heat for the body, on the birth of the baby the mother entered a cold state. The system was never explained to me in this analytical way, and in fact Carol Laderman was able to do so only after talking to a large number of people and getting them to classify the foods. It was clear from my talks with Malay midwives, however, that they accepted this system and used it in their work.

Limah helped women give birth in their own houses and would go over to help as soon as a client called. She said that most women gave birth lying on their back: "I help to keep her body straight so that it will be easy for the baby to come out. If her pain gets very bad we only pray, and sometimes I give her *jampi* betel leaf to reduce the pain." There will usually be a number of relatives around to help. The husband will be nearby, although he won't usually be in the same room in which the birth is taking place unless his wife gets very distressed or is ill: "For three days after the birth I will do the massage and bathe the mother in a special bath made up with the leaves from various plants. [She showed me these plants, most of which were growing like weeds around her house.] She has this in the morning, after which I give her a massage. All this makes the mother feel fresh and good after all the pain she has gone through. After the bath I mix turmeric powder and salt and apply it to her stomach and tie it with a cloth. I do this for three days, to help the stomach return to its flat state. After three days, if the mother wants, I do the *tuku* massage, which is a special massage on the stomach with a metal ball which helps to flatten the stomach. I do it like this: I get a bed which is about three foot high and then I put a small charcoal stove which has been lighted underneath it. Then I ask the woman to lie on the bed in a straight position. Then I heat up the *tuku* ball a little, wrap it in a cloth and push the womb up with it. I do this for fifteen days, and after that I just roll it all around the stomach for a few days."

I decided to have a massage from Limah to see what it was like, and as I lay down the windows and doors were suddenly filled with children come to look at this curious foreigner. Limah started by massaging my legs and said that she would spend a lot of time on the thighs, as this helps the stomach to flatten. She then massaged my stomach quite deeply. After this I sat up while she massaged my back and shoulders, which she said was good for encouraging the milk to flow; I was still breastfeeding, so she showed me how she gently massaged the breasts, one hand above and one hand below each breast to stimulate the flow of milk. She then finished by combing my hair with oil. It certainly felt invigorating, but whether I would have wanted something quite so deep after giving birth I don't know. she said the aim was to "put the women back together again" as well as helping them to feel more energetic – it would certainly do that!

Limah's work had been changed considerably by the government midwife, but she remembered many remedies, some of which she showed us. One of the most interesting was a cure for perineal tears. She poured some special honey (the best being obtained from the Orang Asli in the jungle) in to an earthenware pot and rubbed a special nut into it. This would be put on the tear for several days, and any remainder would be drunk by the woman to help heal internal wounds. For infections of the baby's eyes she said the best thing was to put the mother's milk in them, and she also showed us a remedy for infant colic. This consisted of a type of sea shell which was boiled with the root of one of the common plants, the resulting water being fed to the baby. Unfortunately none of her five daughters was interested in the work, but she was hoping that she might be able to pass on her knowledge to one of her cousins.

Salmah lived just across the way from Limah in a much less imposing house with fewer consumer durables inside it. We thought there was probably some competition between the two midwives, although both strenuously denied this. I think we would have had to be in the kampong for a long time to find out what was really going on between them. Unlike Limah, Salmah had learnt how to be a *bidan* by helping other *bidans* and from picking up what information she could from the government midwife and any other knowledgeable people. For this reason I felt she had far less confidence than Limah, as she had to prove herself entirely from her actions rather than from the fact that she had been initiated by an accepted traditional midwife or a member of her family. In years gone by the ritual aspects of being a *bidan* were far more important than they are now, although all the midwives I spoke to made considerable use of *jampi* or prayers. What was not clear, however, was whether these were Islamic or more magical incantations from the Hindu past. None of the *bidans* was willing to tell me, although it was clear that extensive use was made of the Koran to help women at critical times in the pregnancy and birth process. Because of their ritual expertise in birth, *bidans* used to be employed by the village to plant the first seedlings of rice to ensure that the crop would be prolific. In former times a *bidan* would be engaged at the seventh month of pregnancy and would carry out important rituals to ensure a trouble-free pregnancy and birth. So important was the *bidan* considered to be that the ninety-nine laws of Perak (one of the Malaysian states) compiled during the eighteenth century directed that Muslims should feed the *bidan* of a village along with the district judge, mosque officials and the magician.

Nowadays the position of the traditional midwife is much more equivocal. She is condemned both by the medical establishment for her barbaric practices and insanitary techniques, and by the Islamic religious establishment for contaminating pure Islam with pagan rituals from a Hindu past. As far as her fellow villagers are concerned, however, the *bidan* is a distinguished member of the community, and even middle-class women steeped in Western culture and medicine are likely to ask for her services – if not in giving birth, then for massage and postnatal rituals which are considered necessary. During the long apprenticeship which most traditional midwives have she will learn not only the practical things but also whether she has the right *angin* or spirit to do the work. As one *bidan* told me, "A *bidan* must be brave, as the responsibility of human life rests on her." Whereas the necessary practical expertise can be taught, the *angin* is something that can only be inherited, and becomes apparent only during the apprenticeship with an experienced practitioner. Without such an apprenticeship, the quality of Salmah's *angin* would always be in question. Despite this she had built up quite a following, and she delivered fifteen to twenty babies a year; in fact while we were talking to her a prospective client sat and listened. Like all the *bidans* I talked to, her work had been greatly changed by the coming of the government midwife, and there were now several things which she wasn't allowed to do: "The *missi* [government midwife] must come for the delivery. She delivers the baby, cuts the cord and then goes, leaving me to do all the rest."

Further up the road in the next village, Kampong Tawang, I met Aminah. Here most of the men were fishermen and the women worked at various related jobs such as gutting the fish and pounding it up to make a fish paste. This kampong was noticeably poorer, with smaller and older-looking houses which had much less inside them. Very few people owned any form of mechanical transport such as cars or even motorbikes. I was surprised that two kampongs so close should display such differences in their wealth, but was told this was because the towkay who owned Kampong Tawang took more profits than that of Pemuda, although I never found out whether this was the real reason or not.

Aminah, at fifty, was the youngest Malay *bidan* I talked to and also the busiest, attending five or more births each month. Given that for each birth she looked after the mother for three days as well as providing massage and help for those who were pregnant, it must have been almost a full-time job for her. She also seemed to have the best relationship with the government midwife: "They come and fetch me when the woman is ready to give birth. Some give birth in the house and some in the clinic. They also take me to the clinic because they feel safe when I am around." She was willing to admit that she did quite a few deliveries on her own: "Nowadays the *missi* must be around when a woman is giving birth; but when she is not around – which is sometimes – I'll attend to the delivery alone. So far no one has said anything about me doing this." She was clearly somewhat on edge about her ambivalent status; at first she said that for any difficulties she would send the women to the clinic, but slowly she told us about some of the traditional remedies she still used for things like morning sickness, indigestion, infected eyes, perineal tears, and so on.

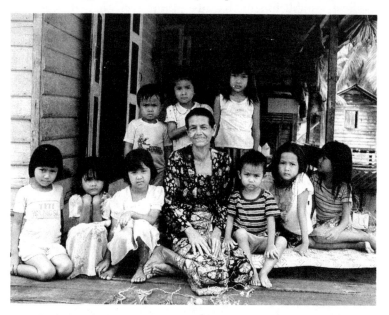

Aminah, a Malay midwife, with some of her family and friends

I asked her about the *pantang*. When I discussed this with some of my Malay friends, the explanation for the restrictions seemed to derive from feeling both that the mother and baby were particularly vulnerable during that time, and that they were somehow not quite clean given that the blood from the birth was still being discharged. None of this, however, was spelled out very clearly to me. Aminah felt that whether one adhered to all the restrictions of the *pantang* or not was a very individual thing: "Some people do observe the *pantang* for forty-four days during which they don't take oily food [as it is thought to make the uterus collapse], cold food [as the mother has entered a 'cold' period] and certain types of fish [thought to exacerbate the cold], but I don't do this. I used to tell my daughters to eat whatever they liked, but if they found that a certain food didn't agree with them to stop taking it for a while. Some adhere to the taboo because they are afraid they will have pain, and others believe in the superstition."

The *pantang* has been roundly criticized by some of the medical establishment because they feel that it leads to inadequate nutrition just when a woman needs to be eating well to recover from the birth and to establish breastfeeding. Carol Laderman found, as I did, that there is considerable individual variation in how much a woman subscribes to the different food restrictions. It is accepted that the prescriptions are merely a guide, and the effects of not following them will depend very much on the health of the mother and her own individual make-up. Carol Laderman found that the nutritional disadvantages were determined by how poor the mother was. Rich mothers could afford the more expensive alternatives to some of the foods which were not allowed and were thus sometimes better nourished during the *pantang* than at other times. Poorer mothers, who were generally less well fed during their pregnancy, could not always afford any reasonable alternatives and could become even more nutritionally deficient at this time. It was not the *pantang* itself which led to nutritional problems but rather the economic situation of the mother.

If, despite the *pantang*, a woman has problems after birth, their is a special postnatal ceremony which a *bomoh* will undertake. I didn't come across this myself, but Carol Laderman did several times during the fifteen months of her stay in the kampong. It is called *main puteri* and is undertaken for any postpartum problems which are generally considered to be psychic in origin rather than physical. In the West we often describe this as postnatal depression. The *bomoh* puts the woman into a trance during which she can express any emotion she likes. Given that Malay society can be very repressive, with little opportunity for outward show of emotion, this can be seen as a way in which "unsuitable" feelings can be expressed and released.

The end of the *pantang* is signified by the ritual introduction to earth, air and water which used to be carried out by the *bidan* for everyone but nowadays is often confined to the babies of the royal families. In its simple form the baby is brought down the steps of the house by the *bidan*, who will put a cross on the baby's feet before putting the feet first on iron, then on a tray containing gold and silver, and lastly on the earth. Thus the baby is introduced to the world, a new mother-and-child unit takes its place in the community, and the *bidan* is discharged from her duties. The baby may then be put for the first time in a cradle into which a cat, a curry stone and a piece of iron will also be placed to terrify evil spirits.

Aminah worked extremely hard and yet, unlike the mid-wives in Kampong Pemuda, felt that she was unable to charge a particular fee for her services: "I don't charge my patients; I accept any amount they care to give – $4 or $5 – whatever they can afford. It is all right even when no money is given, as there is no point in asking them for money when they don't have it. If they have it they will give it to me. I don't demand it because I know they can't afford it." Aminah was held in high esteem by the members of her kampong, but had ambivalent feelings about doing the work: "I don't like being a midwife because it is messy, with all the blood and so on. At first I couldn't eat my food after a delivery, but now I am used to it. I would stop attending to births but the people here want me to carry on, so I continue to do it. It's like helping people and it's one of the reasons why they like me and won't let me leave this place. Even if I say that I want to go to another kampong, they will refuse to let me go!"

To a Malay mother, pregnancy is a normal condition requiring few adjustments in her daily life. Physical activity is believed to facilitate labour, and few changes of diet are required, although too much jackfruit and durian in the early months of pregnancy are not considered a good idea. The reason for this stems both from the traditional ideas about conception and birth and from ideas based on the hot/cold dichotomy. Traditionally the baby is said to be formed in the father's brain, from where it travels to the father's eye and then to his chest, which is considered to be the microcosmic centre of the universe for each person. Here, in the dwelling place of the heart, the baby experiences both the father's rationality and his emotions, after which it descends to the father's penis and is thrust into the mother's womb. This is the baby's resting place where he/she develops and grows and receives his/her mother's earth, air, fire and water until ready for birth. Once the baby has been thrust into the mother's womb, the womb closes to keep the menstrual blood from escaping and further semen from entering. At this time, in the very beginning, the fœtus is considered to be a blood clot and in the early stages anything hot could liquefy the blood and make the womb uncongenial for the child. Hence the dietary restrictions against eating jackfruit and durian, which are considered to be very hot foods. It is interesting that vitamins obtained from the government clinics are sometimes considered equally harmful because they are very "heaty" as well as making the baby grow too big.

Until the fifth month the baby is said to grow "by the grace of God" and to share its mother's soul, so if it is born before the fifth month it will not need to be given an Islamic burial. After the fifth month it is thought to be fed by a conduit from the mother's stomach to the uterus, while air is passed from the mother's lungs to the baby's nose and mouth. As the baby develops it goes hard and soft, and all the Malay *bidans* I spoke to explained it thus: "Usually the baby's head is hard in the seventh month, soft in the eighth month and hard again in the ninth. That is why babies born in the eighth month seldom survive." This, of course, is in direct contradiction to the Western way of looking at things, whereby a baby born one month prematurely would be expected to have a better chance of survival than one born earlier. The placenta, which is thought of as "the baby's little brother", develops during the second month, but as the baby grows he/she moves away from the sibling and hence develops the umbilical cord.

During the pregnancy the baby is considered to be far more at risk than the mother, and there are various mainly symbolic things which the mother and father should do to protect the fœtus and ensure a smooth birth. The father's actions are thought to affect the baby more at the beginning of the pregnancy, with his influence diminishing as the pregnancy progresses and ceasing when the cord is cut after birth. He must kill only animals which are required for food, and must do so cleanly. If he is cutting wood he must make sure that no jagged edges or splinters are left. This is because animals and wood possess quantities of *semangat*, which could harm or disfigure the baby. The concept of *semangat* is an important one for Malays but is difficult for outsiders to conceptualize. It has been described as "the vital force" or "life energy", the energizing power of all things: the energy that makes the rice grow as well as the energy in man. Thus in man *semangat* is a part of the soul, but not the soul itself, and makes its appearance the moment the umbilical cord is severed. After birth the baby's *semangat* has only a precarious hold on its new lodgings, while the mother's has been depleted by her labour. For this reason mother and baby are particularly at risk from spirits and magic that attack their *semangat*, and various measures must be taken to protect them.

One of the easiest ways of doing this is to use stone, iron or nuts, which are thought to have *semangat* in a very concentrated form and thus to scare away any spirits interested in attacking the *semangat* of mother and newborn baby. Within the individual, nail clippings and hair are thought to be particularly dense in *semangat* and one therefore has to be very careful how one disposes of these clippings in case anyone should use them for magical purposes. The first hair cut from a girl baby is thought to be very strong and might be buried at the foot of a barren tree to bring forth fruit "as luxuriant as her tresses". When a person dies the *semangat* dies with the body or may be retained in the shape of a body that wonders around as a *hantu* or ghost.

Most of the things that a couple do to protect the baby before birth, however, will be to stop its *semangat* being affected as well as to ensure an easy and trouble-free labour. A pregnant woman should carry a knife or a piece of iron with her whenever she goes away, as this will harden her and the baby's *semangat* and frustrate evil spirits. After the engagement of the *bidan* during the seventh month the husband should not cut his hair, as this could make the placenta break up; similarly, if the husband goes out at night he should not return directly to his house, but to confuse the evil spirits should take a devious route home. It is also very important that neither husband nor wife obstruct doorways during the pregnancy, as this could obstruct the birth; similarly, pregnant women should not go in one door and out the other, as "there is only one exit to the womb". A pregnant woman should not see anything which is disgusting or distressing, as this could have an effect on the unborn baby, maybe disfiguring him or her in some way. Babies can be described as "fish- ape-, or dog-struck", depending on what the physical deformity resembles in the animal world. These are usually mild deformities, however, as more serious ones cannot be cured and must be seen as a lesson from God.

Despite this seemingly very long list of admonitions, pregnancy is not usually a time of high anxiety, as although doing certain things *can* cause untoward things to happen, the chances are that nothing will happen even if they are. Often they are used much more on an *ex post facto* basis as explanations of why things happened as they did, and sometimes to effect a cure. For example, one mother with a baby who was constantly sick remembered that she had seen a cat being sick while she was pregnant. She therefore got the fur and claws of a cat, which she burnt, and then put the ash on the baby.

A Malay friend of mine – married, as it happens, to an

Englishman – had problems with her baby crying at night soon after he was born. One night, after they'd tried all the soothing things the baby books suggest, and failed, Zam decided that it must be evil spirits. The cure for this was to rub the baby's feet with a mixture of onions and garlic; since the baby fell asleep soon afterwards, Zam was convinced that she was right and took various other measures to protect her baby. One of these was to have a "decontamination" room where anyone who had been outside (especially at night) had to go before being allowed into the rest of the house. This was not the first time I had heard these spirits alluded to, as my maid was once convinced that my daughter had either seen or been attacked by them when she fell ill with a sore throat. The circumstances were rather peculiar and we had thought so at the time, as Emma had gone walking around the house and come running in very suddenly, crying. It is unusual for her to cry without good reason and we could find no reason at all as, unlike her, she continued to cry for some time. When she had seemed to get over it we took her swimming, but after a time she started crying again. Very worried by this time, we took her to a doctor who told us that she had an exceptionally bad sore throat. My maid did not deny the existence of the sore throat, but saw it as a symptom of the illness caused by the spirits rather than the cause of the illness itself.

Most people I talked to were very vague about the spirits and couldn't – or wouldn't – tell me much about them. There are, however, a number of spirits which are thought to attack mothers and babies in particular; these include the *bajong*, which takes the form of the pole cat; the *langsuit*, which takes the form of an owl with long claws; and the *pontianak* or *mati anak*, which is also a form of night owl. Perhaps the most horrible is the *penanggulan*, which resembles a trunkless human being with her entrails hanging out; she is said to fly about seeking the opportunity to suck the blood out of babies. Many of these spirits – but the last in particular – are thought to emanate from women who have died in childbirth. This is why, when this happens, glass beads will be put in the corpse's mouth to stop her screaming, hens' eggs will be put under her armpits to stop her flying, and needles put into the palms of her hands so that she can't open and close them to assist her in the flight. Another spirit, called the spirit of the earth [*jin tanah*] or the black genie [*jin hitam*], is attracted to the blood of parturition which may drip through the floorboards of traditional houses to the earth below.

Much of what the traditional midwife used to do was involved with keeping these spirits away with the use of charms, amulets like iron and stone, and maybe thorned branches under the floor of the house. She would also make sure that the woman was in the most appropriate place for birth and facing the "right" way – all of which would depend on the heat or cold of the woman's body, the time of day, and so on, and would therefore be individually determined for each client by the *bidan*.

In my talks with these *bidans*, the government midwife – or *missi*, as she was known locally – featured prominently in their conversations. It was difficult, during the short time I had to talk to them, to explore in any detail the relationship between themselves and the government authorities. It is very difficult indeed to discuss any sort of antagonism between organizations or individuals openly in this society, as there is a strong feeling towards consensus and any splits tend to be covered up or not openly acknowledged, especially to outsiders. Everyone I spoke to maintained that they had a good relationship with the government midwife and wouldn't discuss it in any detail. Carol Laderman was extremely lucky in this respect, as living in such a community for over a year gave her a chance to look at this relationship in detail and see how it was acted out.

A government midwife in Malaysia has a training of two years in a hospital, where she has to attend at least thirty women in labour and witness no fewer than twenty deliveries. This is in contrast to the traditional midwives who, in the village where Carol Laderman stayed, had all been in practice for thirty years or more after a long apprenticeship with their mothers or other female relatives. To the villagers the government midwife was a stranger and, being paid by the government, usually a very rich stranger by comparison with themselves. While they respected her official authority, command of scientific apparatus and medicines and the ability to call an ambulance in times of difficulty, she was still considered a foreigner and did not have the trust inspired by the village *bidans*. This was exacerbated by various aspects of the *missi's* work. Unlike the *bidan*, whom one could call or go and see at any time if difficulties were experienced, the government midwife had clinics for which appointments had to be made, whether one felt the need or not.

The ambivalence towards the government midwife intensified over the issue of whether or not she would actually be there for the birth. With her clinic, her other work and the large geographical area she had to cover (in which six traditional midwives worked) the government midwife was always pushed for time to carry out all her necessary duties. When a woman went into labour she would call the government midwife, who would come in time or not, depending on where she was in the district and what else she was doing. If it looked as if the mother might be some time before giving birth she would have to estimate when the baby was likely to be born, and in the light of that decide whether to leave and get on with her other work. On many occasions the government midwife made the wrong decision and was not there when the baby was born.

Traditional midwives also had to make similar decisions, as they had other work to do which often took them away from the village. Whereas the government midwife was seen as very unreliable in this respect, the traditional midwives, by contrast, were seen as extremely reliable; in the months Carol Laderman spent in the village, not one mistake was made by any of the *bidans*, who were always there when the baby was born – this presumably being the result of their greater practical experience. The government midwife, however, was crucial in an emergency, as it was only she who could send for the ambulance to take a woman to hospital. There was a strong feeling amongst the villagers that it was therefore necessary to register with the government midwife so that she was available to perform this service should it be required. While the government midwife advised birth in hospital, this was not acceptable to most women, who saw hospital as a place for sick people. While they were aware that danger could arise from an ordinary pregnancy, they preferred to take a "wait and see" attitude, as experience had shown them that in most cases everything went all right.

The midwives I spoke to said they rarely experienced problems and I wondered if maybe they were unwilling to admit to any, as this might reflect badly on them. I was told, however, that even in the very worst cases, where the mother or baby died, this wouldn't necessarily be seen as the *bidan's* fault. Rather, it would be seen as the time decreed by Allah for the mother or baby to go to Him. Thus, provided the *bidan* had used all the practical and spiritual means at her disposal, she would be absolved from any blame. Whatever the problems she was faced with, she was always able to summon spiritual help. Carol Laderman found that a *bidan* in difficulties might turn to the local *bomoh* for help, which he would provide in the form of mythological chanting. She looked at some of these chants and found that they put the labour pains into a meaningful context, with the promised satisfactory ending of a baby. Thus, however unproductive and chaotic labour might feel to the mother, this chanting would help to show her that this was not the case. The *bomoh* might also identify the woman's reproductive powers with universal creativity, using symbols to focus on the drama of birth.

Whatever he did it would be the woman who retained the central role – unlike in the West, where the doctor would feel that he would have to take over. In the West, pregnancy and birth are viewed as constituting a potentially life-threatening illness, so that the mother must be placed in the hands of an obstetrician whose decision is final. Pregnancy and birth may, of course, imperil the well-being of the Malay mother, but such dangers are considered very rare, and even if they did occur they would not be allowed to erode her autonomy. Whatever a mother's decision, it would not be questioned by either the family or the *bidan*; she is the labouring mother and it is she who knows what is best for herself and her baby. This gives the Malay mother a tremendous and maybe, to our Western eyes, awesome responsibility; as Carol Laderman puts it, "American women are delivered of babies by the obstetrician; Malay women give birth." How long will it be before this changes?

Already, as we have seen, women are being strongly encouraged to give birth in hospitals, many of which provide the worst of what Western medicine has to offer, with a conveyor-belt mentality and routine intervention. Traditional midwives are denigrated by the authorities, and the important service they provide for poorer mothers in rural areas is not recognized. It grieves me greatly to see this tradition being thrown away when we in the West are now trying to revive it: finding ways to support the natural process of birth rather than ways to control it.

POSTSCRIPT

12

⏳

FURTHER THOUGHTS:

THROUGHOUT MY TRAVELS and in the course of collecting this information I could not help comparing the experiences of the mothers and midwives to whom I had spoken with my own experience of birth. Perhaps the first thing I was always aware of was the extent to which I had been able to choose, not only when I would have a child but also whether I would ever have any children or not. For many of the women in these traditional societies, bearing and rearing children was as inevitable as the sun rising and setting each day. It was part of their unquestioned identity as a woman even when, like the Orang Asli, they felt they had some control over the matter. I became pregnant after a considerable amount of thought and agonizing about whether this was what I wanted to do and whether I could cope with the changes it would bring in my life. The women I spoke to became pregnant in the fullness of time as part of what they considered to be the natural order of things over which, on the whole, they felt they had very little control.

Having made the choice and eventually become pregnant, I naturally turned to the institutional provision which we have for pregnancy and birth in the West. Unlike most of the women I spoke with I had never seen a baby being born and had never helped with a birth, in spite of growing up in an unusually large family. For information I turned to books rather than my mother or other female relatives. This was partly because I wanted to be as up to date as possible and I thought their experiences would be out of date, and partly because this was something my mother and I had never discussed, and it never occurred to me to do so. This contrasted greatly with so many of the groups I visited where things change very slowly and mothers consider that teaching their daughters about how to give birth is one of the most important things they do. In any case, like so many women in the West, by the time I became pregnant I was living a long way away from any relatives who could have provided practical help.

Not unnaturally, I felt a strong responsibility towards my unborn baby and wanted to do the very best for her. At this time the "very best" meant regular attendance at antenatal checkups and arranging to have my baby in the safety of a hospital. The problem was that I found the antenatal checkups more upsetting than reassuring and I began to question whether they were really as good and necessary for the health of myself and my baby as the medical profession assured me they were. Having a first baby at the age of twenty-nine put me in a "high-risk" category which seemed to limit the choices I had over where and how I gave birth. I managed to persuade my general practitioner to provide some of my antenatal care, but she did so very reluctantly and antenatal checkups became even more of a trial. Every time I saw her she reiterated all the problems I could expect to encounter because of my age, and why a home birth was therefore impossible. Perhaps if I had been a little older, more confident in my feelings and more assertive, I could have coped with this situation more creatively. But having been led to believe that giving birth to a baby was a medical problem with medical answers, I was very ambivalent about not conforming to these ideas. My GP was extremely gratified when I finally developed high blood pressure, thus vindicating what she had always said and providing a cast-iron excuse for referral to a hospital.

I shall never forget my first visit to the hospital and in particular my conversation with the consultant who, I had been assured, was one of the better ones with some idea about the psychological aspects of labour and birth. As usual, I had been prepared for his ministrations by a nurse and was lying ready for his examination. I can't remember his exact words, but I can remember how I felt belittled by his cursory dismissal of how I said I wanted my birth to be. Lying there with no clothes on while he prodded around and gave me all the usual arguments for the superiority of his way of doing things, I became totally demoralized and felt that the very strong emotions I had about what was right for me and my unborn baby were somehow wrong. Perhaps his parting shot was the worst of all – "You want to have a healthy baby, don't you?" – leaving the unspoken assumption that the only way to achieve this was to do as he said, and that if I didn't then it would all be my fault. It was only much, much later that I realized how I had been coerced into losing my autonomy and to giving responsibility to the doctor rather than taking it for myself.

Not surprisingly, things did get worse and eventually I was admitted to hospital, which had a nightmarish quality that even after all these years I can hardly bear to think about. What I felt I needed to help both my blood pressure and my emotional state was a room on my own with peace and quiet; but this was denied on the grounds that there were only a few such rooms and I was not ill enough to be allocated one. Once again I became totally demoralized and unsure about my own feelings of what was right for me. I was given drugs; there didn't seem any way to avoid them, as once I had got into the system it ground on with a horrible inevitability and I became even more upset and ill. I suppose the birth could have been worse – but at least I was awake when Mary was born, and this did make up to some extent for the epidural and the forceps delivery. Even then, the doctor felt Mary had to be taken away to special care, which of course was two floors above the ward in which I was staying.

Once I had Mary, who was alive and well, the hospital

arguments with which I had been coerced to do things "for the baby's sake" no longer had any force. I felt I could do as I liked and went up to the nursery whenever I felt like it, fed Mary at all hours and got myself a single room, which was easier to arrange postnatally. I know there must be many women who have had similar and worse experiences but it took me many, many years to some to terms with the resulting anger and alienation that I had felt from being denied the support and consideration for my feelings as a person.

Some would argue, of course, that I was very lucky and that if I had been a woman in, say, a Minangkabau or a Karen village I would probably have been at best very ill or at worst dead. I can't help wondering, however, to what extent my high blood pressure and other problems were exacerbated by the system. If I had not had the negative feedback from my GP, if I had had my real needs at least acknowledged and dealt with sympathetically by the hospital, if I had stood more by my own feelings of what I needed, would I have had all those problems? That, of course, I can never know, although I think it was significant that the one time a doctor did acknowledge my feelings, my blood pressure went down for the next twenty-four hours. In any of the traditional villages I visited I would have received far more support from family, friends and the midwife, who would know and understand my feelings, than I received from anyone in the hospital.

One of the things I continually thought about on my travels was whether the midwives and mothers I spoke to had anything to say to us in the West. Most of the time I was very divided about this and swung between feeling that the yawning gaps in lifestyle could never be bridged and yet also experiencing a tremendous affinity with most of those women. Obviously we cannot return to pre-industrial ways of living and the integrated lifestyles that go with it, neither would most people want to. Also the spiritual context, which is often so important in these societies, cannot be transported from the society in which it is embedded.

Having said that, however, I feel that the setting in which

traditional midwives operate is so much more wholesome than what we have in the West. Birth in the West is divorced from everyday life, is hidden away in hospitals and is something mothers go through very discreetly, and then emerge with a baby tied up in nice clothes to be duly admired by the rest of the family and friends. This is the extreme, of course, and the home birth movement, active birth and radical midwives are a very necessary and hopeful reaction to this situation. Whatever our differences, however, we are talking about an experience shared by women everywhere, although it is interpreted in so many different ways even in the relatively small part of the world in which I have travelled. Perhaps what these women have to tell us is that the way we deal with birth in the West is but one way. Knowing there are other ways can point us towards the benefits and limitations of our own system, and in so doing give us more choice as to how we give birth ourselves.

I an often asked how effective traditional midwives really are, and whether they do a good job or cause more problems than they prevent. I am not a qualified medical practitioner and I did not have the resources to carry out the sort of research necessary to answer such questions definitively. The more midwives I saw and talked to, however, the more I was struck by their dedication and their desire to do the best they could for the women who came to them for help. Without exception they all had a tremendous range of experience; most had borne children of their own and served a long apprenticeship before they began practising. One of their big advantages is that they share the same ideas and the spiritual and practical life of the mothers for whom they give their services so freely, and they usually know these mothers well. Whatever help the traditional midwife gives is always given according to what the mother feels she needs, and her autonomy is rarely questioned or compromised.

Traditional midwives usually have some spiritual calling for their work, which gives them and their clients confidence in their ability to deal with both normal and abnormal births. They use techniques which are appropriate to their situation:

bamboo is a good thing to use for cutting the umbilical cord in communities which neither understand nor have the facilities for sterilizing instruments. In every group I visited there were simple, cheap and easily available remedies for most of the common problems associated with pregnancy and birth. I would say, therefore, that they are as good as anyone at dealing with normal births [I would include breech babies in that category] and a good deal better than many in the way they work with the mothers. I saw little evidence that their practices would actually cause problems. Often I thought that using massage, which is so central to traditional midwifery practice, was very beneficial and could usefully be copied by midwives in the West.

Traditional midwives can't, of course, deal with serious cases that might need surgical intervention, but how many such cases are there? I have come across various estimates, ranging from 5 per cent to as high as 15 per cent, but of course this is usually based on figures from developed countries, where it is difficult to say how much of this intervention is strictly necessary. Even with the higher estimate, however, I think that a traditional midwife could deal extremely well with the vast majority of births. There are, of course, other problems which a traditional midwife might not recognize and even if she did, might not be able to do anything about. Someone working in Somalia, for instance, found that the traditional midwives did not recognize pre-eclampsia; or rather, they recognized it but, as they had no treatment for it, ignored it and hoped that God would provide the necessary help. Once shown how they could alleviate this condition, however, they were only too pleased to do so.

Many people dismiss completely the traditional beliefs and magical practices which many of these practitioners and their clients consider is the most important part of their work as no more than superstition. Most of what they do, however, is to support the woman in her own experience of labour and birth. There is a lot of research which shows how intimately body and mind are connected. To what extent do these beliefs support the mind, so helping the body to function better? To what extent do the symbolic things which a woman does during pregnancy – such as not obstructing doorways, and so on – help to bring her awareness to the need for her body to open and allow the baby to be born? Those who view the body as no more than a physical vehicle like a car will not, of course, accept such ideas. But there are many women who have found that images, which either consciously or unconsciously arise, can be very helpful.

In giving birth, women can go into a state of what is sometimes described as "non-ordinary reality", which is the state which shamans and other spiritual healers are said to enter and from which they derive their healing powers. In the West this state of being is usually discounted, although there are a few people who are beginning to realize its potential and are learning how to use it both to maintain health and to help cure illness. In so many of the places I visited this state of "non-ordinary reality" was very important, and of course the traditional midwife was the expert in this as far as giving birth was concerned. I think that many women who have been able to have a natural and uninterrupted birth in the West have entered this state spontaneously (as I did myself during my second birth) and have been able to use the power it provides to give birth successfully. Rather than concentrating on even more "hi-tech" gadgets with which to control birth, we should be looking at these equally powerful internal forces which we have at our disposal and which in the West we have hardly tapped at all.

The decline in neonatal deaths in many Third World countries has sometimes been explained in terms of the superior, usually Western-type, medical systems which have been instituted. While this may be true to some extent, for many of the people I talked to the lowering of the neonatal death rate had more to do with better food and clean water than with more antenatal checkups. In many developing countries the cost of setting up a Western-type medical system is very high, and many do not have the resources to run one adequately. Often health services are concentrated in hospitals, which tend to be in towns, so health provision in rural areas is much worse. Where private medicine is allowed to flourish, the gap between the medical care of the rich and the poor can be extremely wide. At the same time, traditional medical systems are at best unsupported and at worst undermined, so that they gradually die out, leaving the poor with no or very inadequate care.

In Malaysia, for instance, traditional midwives are not allowed to cut the umbilical cord and a government midwife must be called in to do it. This apparently simple rule has given the authorities a way of controlling traditional midwives while at the same time undermining their methods which, as far as I know, have never been researched to see whether they are really as bad for mothers as the conventional doctors make out. In rural areas there are not enough government midwives to provide the necessary care, so a blind eye is turned to the traditional midwives who fill in the gaps, especially as far as aftercare is concerned. With their ambivalent status, however, traditional midwives are rarely passing on their knowledge to others, and in the next thirty years or so will probably more or less disappear, leaving only a very inadequate system in their place. I think it is very ironic that whereas in the West we are realizing the importance of – and in some cases turning back to – holistic ways of curing illness and giving birth, in developing countries the holistic system which they already have is so often disappearing.

The so-called improvements in maternity provision have often been bought at a terrible price for mothers and their newborn babies. With scarce resources, hospitals are built and run with only the physical rather than the psychological and emotional needs of patients in mind. For mothers expecting babies, this means crowded antenatal clinics, inadequate provision for family support, and a conveyor-belt attitude towards birth, with routine intervention. I visited a hospital in the town where I lived in Malaysia and was shown the labour ward. It consisted of four beds in a row on which lay four women, on their backs (physiologically the worst position in which to give birth), two of whom had drips in their arms. There was one nurse on duty and none of the women was allowed to have anyone with her for support or comfort. What I found unnerving was the total silence that prevailed – it was more like a place of death than one of giving life. This place was not exceptional, and in fact the doctor who showed me round was very proud of the modern facilities and the way in which he "managed" labour, which he thought was a big improvement for women. Private medicine tends to increase the amount of intervention and Caesarean deliveries, the ultimate in labour management and an excellent way of making money, become ever more common.

For me, the culmination of this work has been in the changes in my own attitudes to my third pregnancy. I have focused far more upon myself and have drawn more security from my feelings about what is happening rather than from the tests the doctor does. This pregnancy has been a wonderful learning process about how to find and keep the security of the knowledge and feelings in my centre, when all around me doctors are only too willing to take away my autonomy and my responsibility. I thought at first that I wouldn't be able to finish this book until I'd given birth and perhaps shown that I had "successfully" done so with my new-found knowledge and insights. Thinking about it, however, I've realized that whatever happens is in some ways less important than the way I respond to it, and that to define "success" in any particular way before giving birth is to miss the point of the experience. I look forward with excitement and wonder to the miracle of giving birth again.

BIBLIOGRAPHY

I used a wide variety of academic articles and general books and papers to supplement my impressions and fill the gaps in my knowledge. I found that very little had been written on the subject of traditional midwives in this part of the world. By far the best and most informative is *Wives and Midwives* by Carol Laderman (University of California Press, 1983). Laderman spent fifteen months living in a Malay kampong and helping the traditional midwives with their work, as well as investigating local ideas about nutrition during pregnancy and after birth. She gives a wonderfully detailed insight into the work of these traditional practitioners.

Other books about Malaysia included:

Malay Magic by William Skeat, first printed in 1899 and reprinted by Oxford University Press in 1984. William Skeat was an English civil servant in what was then Malaya who collected data about the Malay magical practices he saw. This book has an interesting account of beliefs about childbirth.

Orang Asli by Iskander Carey (Oxford University Press, 1976). An account of the different Orang Asli groups in Malaysia by someone who was head of the Department of Orang Asli Affairs for some years.

An introduction to the different hill tribes of Thailand can be found in *The Hill Tribes of Thailand* (Tribal Research Institute of Chang Mai University, 1986). This small institute has a library from which I obtained many articles about the different hill tribe groups I visited.

I obtained information about Indonesia from a wide range of different sources, many of them local, such as: *Minangkabau Culture* by Syamsul Azhar (Topic Printing, Bukittinggi, Indonesia, 1988); *Life and Death in Toraja* by Dr Stanislaus Sandarupa (CV Tiga Taurus, Ujung Pandang, Sulawesi, Indonesia).

GLOSSARY

Adat: customs or traditions. Often behaviour is explained as "part of our *adat*", meaning the traditional way of doing things.

Akar kayu: a general name for medicine made from a mixture of roots and herbs. There are all sorts of akar kayu for different conditions, each practitioner having his or her own mixtures. Most Malay traditional midwives have one for use during pregnancy and after.

Aluk: a word used by the Toraja for a blend of the religious and the practical "right way of living".

Angin: this has many shades of meaning; it can refer to humours within the body, flatulence, or a talent or predisposition towards certain sorts of behaviour.

Attap: a local palm, the leaves of which are used to make houses and roofs.

Baitong: a Torajan spirit who lives a normal family life during the day but at night changes into an evil spirit.

Balai: refers to a community building. *Balai polis*, for instance, is the local police station. In Minangkabau villages it is the community hall where the young men of the village sleep.

Banguin-banguin: a herb used by Batek women to help lactation.

Batin: the headman of a village in Malaysia.

Bersanding: a Malay wedding festival. The couple become "king and queen" for a day. They dress in royal clothes and sit on a dais while friends and relatives come and give them blessings.

Bidan: Malay word for the traditional midwife.

205

Blakho: herb used by the Karen to stop bleeding after childbirth.

Bomoh: Malay traditional doctor experienced in curing all illnesses, using both physical and supernatural means.

Datu: male Batek priests who are specialists in occult knowledge.

Deata: the Gods of the Toraja, who are placed between the Higher Gods and the ancestors, and to whom one gives offerings and prays for help.

Denguin: leaves used by Orang Asli midwives to cleanse themselves after helping with birth.

Dukun: another name for a *bomoh*.

Durian: a large fruit which has a very distinctive smell and taste and is very much prized throughout Malaysia.

Farang: Thai name for a foreigner.

Jampi: prayers, but often refers to the special incantations used by *bidans* and *bomohs*.

Gambir: a sour white paste chewed with betel leaf.

Kebangunun and *kelimau* – plants used by Orang Asli women after they have given birth to strengthen and protect against urinary infection.

Losman: low-cost places for travellers to stay.

Missi: the name given by local Malays to the Government midwife.

Padi: unhusked rice.

Pantang: means literally "prohibited by custom", but often used to refer to the food restrictions that Malay and many Indonesian women adhere to after giving birth.

Penghulu: another name for the headman or *batin*.

Puja: the Toraja afterworld.

Puloi: a root used by the Karen which is made into a tea and drunk by women after giving birth if they are bleeding.

Semangat or *sumangat*: life force or embodied spirit.

Sirih: another name for *betel*, which is chewed throughout Indonesia and Malaysia.

Tondi: Batek word for a person's soul substance.

Tabua: a large ceremonial drum used by the Minangkabau as a warning and signal for meetings; now used mainly to show when the fast of Ramadan begins and ends each day.

INDEX

208

ABOUT THE AUTHOR

JACQUELINE VINCENT-PRIYA has a doctorate in sociology from the University of Surrey. During the four years that she spent in Malaysia she was a regular contributor to the Singaporean magazine *Motherhood* and to various Malaysian magazines and newspapers, including *Medical Management* and *New Straits Times*. She has three children.